APHRODISIACS

AN A–Z

LINDA LOUISA DELL

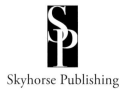

Skyhorse Publishing

Skyhorse Publishing books may be purchased in bulk at special discounts for sales promotion, corporate gifts, fund-raising, or educational purposes. Special editions can also be created to specifications. For details, contact the Special Sales Department, Skyhorse Publishing, 307 West 36th Street, 11th Floor, New York, NY 10018 or info@skyhorsepublishing.com.

Skyhorse® and Skyhorse Publishing® are registered trademarks of Skyhorse Publishing, Inc.®, a Delaware corporation.

Visit our website at www.skyhorsepublishing.com.

10 9 8 7 6 5 4 3 2 1

Library of Congress Cataloging-in-Publication Data is available on file.

Cover design by Jane Sheppard
Cover photo credit: Thinkstock

Print ISBN: 978-1-63220-481-3
Ebook ISBN: 978-1-63220-800-2

Printed in China

To lovers everywhere: Be safe, be strong, and be true to yourself.

WARNING AND DISCLAIMER

In this book I have tried to give information relating to sexuality, sexual problems, and sexual dysfunction that will help people who have suffered from sexual problems or low libido. Making love can be a beautiful and natural experience to be enjoyed and appreciated, but sometimes problems arise that can spoil our enjoyment.

In this book I have listed many aphrodisiacs from the bizarre to the mundane, some of which can help with sexual problems. But I have to stress that much of the information given is intended for curiosity only and that the effects of some herbs, plants, and essential oils can be dangerous, as what is a safe dose for one person can be very toxic for another. The author and publisher can take no responsibility for the misuse of any of the preparations listed herein. The information given is not intended to take the place of medical advice and attention.

Contents

CHAPTER ONE

An Introduction to Sex Drive and Libido

Low sex drive is very common and can affect up to one-fifth of the population at any one time. In researching this book, I was astonished at the enormous range of aphrodisiac substances, vitamins, minerals, herbs, essential oils, and drugs that have, reputedly, a profound and beneficial effect on the libido. Jungians often use the name of the Greek god Eros as well as the Latin term *libido* to talk about love energy. By this term they mean not just sexual appetites, but a general appetite for life.

Sex drive, or libido, is more often than not the strongest urge in humans after food and sleep. But all too often, one partner ends up having a lower sex drive than another partner, who can end up feeling frustrated, neglected, or unloved.

Loss of sex drive is extremely common and is now the biggest single reason for consulting a sex therapist. A normal sex drive is needed, as your sexual health and general well-being are very closely linked. Just as the healthier you are, the more you are likely to want to have sex, increased sexual energy is also beneficial to the mind, body, and spirit.

The benefits of regular sex have been recommended throughout the ages. In ancient China, the flow of sexual energy around the body was believed to form the basis of physical, emotional, and spiritual well-being; channeling sexual energy was considered the key to immortality. Herbal aphrodisiacs and erotic arts were therefore used not to increase simply pleasure in sex, but also as a means to advance general health and longevity.

The Greek physician Galen wrote in the second century AD that sexual abstinence was the direct cause of hysteria. In the 1940s, psychoanalyst Wilhelm Reich advocated "an orgasm a day for optimum health." Many researchers have found numerous beneficial effects of indulging in regular sex. The French call sexual climax the "little death," as it may help to postpone that eventual "big death."

In men, male hair growth seems to increase when sex is anticipated, probably as a result of increased testosterone activity. In both men and women, levels of the hormone oxytocin peak during orgasm, have a tranquilizing effect on both sexes, and help to provide a good night's sleep, although the effect appears to be greater in men than in women.

The sex drive, or libido, is a powerful directing force that has a profound effect on human behavior. The term "libido" was first used by the psychoanalyst Sigmund Freud to signify the instinctive psychosexual energy that is present in everyone from birth.

Men are said to reach their sexual peak in their teens, while their psychological sex drive peaks after the age of fifty when testosterone levels fall. Women are said to reach their physical sexual peak in their thirties or forties, while their psychological sex drive reaches its maximum in their fifties, at the same time as that of males. But this is not to say that men and women cannot continue having and enjoying sex up to almost any age.

Losing interest in sex

Even in a settled, loving, long-term relationship, the sensual thrills that accompanied the first flush of love will recede once the passionate honeymoon phase is over. Lovemaking often becomes less exciting and even boring.

Try to keep interest in sex alive by experimenting with different positions and techniques and varying the time and place of lovemaking so your love life does not become stale. There can be many reasons for sex drive to fall or fail; these can include medical or lifestyle situations such as:

- Familiarity or boredom
- Being unfit or overweight or having low self-esteem
- Stress and lack of sleep
- Poor diet or excess alcohol and drugs
- Pregnancy and breastfeeding
- Anxiety or depression
- Pain or illness
- Menopause
- Impotence
- Male menopause, prostate problems, or hypogonadism
- Previous sexual abuse or relationship problems
- SAD (Seasonal Affective Disorder)
- Cultural influences or parents' attitude to sex

Familiarity or boredom

It may be that you are in a loving relationship, but things have gotten a bit predictable. If this is the case, try to bring some excitement back into your relationship. Surprise your partner, try different positions, use sex aids, learn how to massage each other, take a romantic break together, and, if you have children, get someone to look after them at least once a week so you can just concentrate on each other and indulge yourselves without fear of interruptions.

BEING UNFIT OR OVERWEIGHT OR HAVING LOW SELF-ESTEEM

General unfitness, lack of exercise, being overweight, and not liking the way you look can certainly lower sex drive. The first thing to remember is that sex is excellent exercise; you can lose between two hundred and five hundred calories in an average-to-spirited sex session.

In today's society, more people are becoming overweight, which leads to sluggishness and low energy levels, which in turn lead to lack of self-esteem and low sex drive. One of the most inhibiting factors when it comes to making love is lack of confidence in your body shape. It is important for you to love your body, love yourself, and always make your partner feel comfortable with his or her body image and sexuality.

STRESS AND LACK OF SLEEP

Stress is one of the most common causes of loss of libido along with overwork, exhaustion, and lack of sleep. Reducing stress levels will help to boost sex drives in both men and women. You should also aim to avoid coffee, strong tea, caffeinated drinks, cigarettes, and alcohol when you are under stress, as these only make matters worse.

POOR DIET OR EXCESS ALCOHOL AND DRUGS

It is generally estimated that one in ten people do not get all the nutrients they need from their food alone and should take vitamin supplements to complement their diet. I would guess the actual number would be even higher than that.

Alcohol in small quantities is an aphrodisiac, but only for women. Prolonged use of alcohol may hinder men from getting erections. Milk thistle can help to protect liver cells from the effects of alcohol and may boost testosterone levels that have been lowered by excess alcohol intake. Alcohol heightens our feelings and lowers our inhibitions, but too much alcohol dampens the sexual urge and impedes performance. Many commonly prescribed drugs, and some illicit drugs, have a negative effect on sex drive. If you think your low sex drive is linked to a medication you are taking, consult your doctor, but do not stop taking medication except under medical supervision.

Pregnancy and breastfeeding

The effect of pregnancy on one's sex drive varies, as every woman and every pregnancy is different. Psychological influences play a large part, as does increased blood flow to the genital area. Increased lubrication means that orgasm is usually easier to achieve and more intense during pregnancy.

If low sex drive occurs, it is to do with levels of the libido-neutralizing hormone prolactin. After childbirth, the female sex drive will normally return, but sometimes when a woman is breast-feeding, high levels of prolactin will inhibit sexual feelings. This is a way of nature, preventing the woman from becoming pregnant again while her newborn is still very much dependent on her.

Other factors that may affect postnatal sex drive include being sore from stitches or being over-stretched during childbirth as well as low self-esteem, anxiety, and body image. If low sex drive is linked with postnatal depression, you must seek medical help immediately.

Anxiety or depression

Anxiety or depression can lead to physical and emotional exhaustion and loss of sex drive. Depression can be caused by many things, including lifestyle changes, bereavement, illness, or menopause. Always seek medical advice for depression and prolonged anxiety, whatever the cause.

PAIN OR ILLNESS

Physical discomfort when making love can lead to lack of interest or aversion to sex. Pain when making love may be superficial due to vaginal thrush, allergies, cystitis, vaginal dryness, pelvic inflammatory disease, or sexually transmitted diseases. It can also come from pain in the hips, legs, or back. In these cases, care must be taken to find the correct positions that do not put stress on those limbs.

Many long-term diseases, such as those affecting the heart, can lead to loss of sex drive. Some sexual activity helps with a feel-good factor even with long-term illness, but let your doctor be your guide here.

MENOPAUSE

Menopause is a natural time in a woman's life when her fertility draws to an end. It can affect women in two ways: relief and a new sexual freedom or remorse at the loss of a fertile body. The clitoris sometimes becomes less sensitive after menopause, which is probably the main cause of difficulty reaching orgasm at this time. Using a lubricant can help with a dry vagina, which can be uncomfortable during intercourse.

IMPOTENCE

Impotence is the inability to perform sexually due to failure to achieve an erection. There can be many causes for this, either physical or emotional. The word impotence is derived from the Latin *impotentia*, literally "lack of power." The first clinical definition appears in Copland's 1832 *A Dictionary of Practical Medicine*.

MALE MENOPAUSE, PROSTATE PROBLEMS, OR HYPOGONADISM

Male menopause is a time when men experience a lowering of the libido due to the fall in testosterone levels in the body. Prostate and urethra problems can also be a factor. Hypogonadism means functional failure of ovaries or testes, which is caused by underactivity of the hypothalamus and pituitary glands and high prolactin levels. Male hypogonadism results in low sex drive and fertility problems.

PREVIOUS SEXUAL ABUSE OR RELATIONSHIP PROBLEMS

Low sex drive can result from relationship problems, where someone has simply fallen out of love with their partner and is no longer attracted to them, for example. Unresolved anger, abuse, and infidelity can also play an important role, especially when the couple finds it difficult to communicate. Previous sexual abuse can carry over into a current relationship. Where this is a problem, professional counseling may be needed.

SAD (SEASONAL AFFECTIVE DISORDER)

SAD, depression related to changes in seasons, seems to have a dampening effect on the sex drive. Sunlight affects the pineal gland in the brain, promoting desire and the readiness to mate. Many people find they feel sexier in hot, sunny weather.

CULTURAL INFLUENCES OR PARENTS' ATTITUDE TO SEX

Cultural attitudes to sex vary around the world and can have a profound effect on sex drive. In homes where sex is frowned on, parents are overly discreet about their sexual activity or never discuss sex, or where there is a non-sexually active single parent raising a child, a low libido may become the normal role model. This can have a subliminal effect on a child's own sexual attitudes in later life.

Negative social conditioning about sex inevitably creates fear, which is passed from generation to generation by sometimes well-intentioned agents such as parents, teachers, or religious leaders. Fear also inhibits communication in sex so that instead of being a deep communion between two people, lovemaking often becomes a tense encounter in which both partners are afraid to express their real needs.

The reduction of sex to a purely physical act also promotes an externalized idea of intercourse, in which lovemaking is perceived as a performance. "Did you come yet?" an anxious lover may ask. In some religions, sex is considered only an act of procreation.

We must release our inhibitions and allow ourselves to enjoy sex just for the sake of it. Sex should be fun, self-pleasure is not a sin, and sexuality is a vital part of all our lives.

CHAPTER TWO

An Introduction to Aphrodisiacs and Sexual Practices

APHRODISIACS IN HISTORY

Probably the first recorded reference to aphrodisiacs comes from undated Egyptian medical papyri believed to be from the Middle Kingdom, which flourished between 2200 and 1700 BCE. Aphrodisiacs are mentioned in countless volumes of the world's sacred texts. Ancient narratives are filled with glowing accounts of aphrodisiac foods and potions. By the time of the golden age of Greece, their use was fairly commonplace. The Romans were also intimately familiar with the art of culinary seduction and the use of oils and perfumes. Aphrodisiac lore passed from the Roman to the early Christian era, through the Middle Ages and the Renaissance, and to modern times.

PHEROMONES

The sense of vision is strongest in humans, but the sense of smell is dominant in animals and aids survival, communication, sexual attraction, and mating. Apparently the female moth releases a mating pheromone that can be detected by the feathery antennae of the male from over one mile away. However, smell is also important in human mating, as we all release pheromones.

The word pheromone is derived from the Greek *pherin*, "to bring or transfer to," and *hormone*, "to excite." These are manufactured by the apocrine sweat glands and are dotted around the body. When we emit pheromones, they are detected by other people unconsciously and either attract others to or repel others from us. This may be the basis of perfumery. Aromatic oils were and still are used in seduction since aroma is linked with the idea of survival of the species. If odor bypasses the cortex and goes straight to the brain's limbic system, concerned with emotion, our response to an odor is often immediate and instinctive. Perhaps this is why we desire someone or how we fall in love and cannot explain it: we get pleasure from the other person's own personal smell.

It has long been suspected that pheromones play a role in human sexual behavior. As a result, many expensive perfumes have included secretions from the sexual glands of the musk deer, anal glands of the civet cat, and intestine of the sperm whale. These are repellent in their natural states but add a warmer, seductive note to perfumes in miniscule doses and stabilize more fleeting aromas.

Human pheromones are now known to be secreted in small amounts in skin oils around the nipples, under the armpits, and in the genital area. Evolution designed us to secrete pheromones when we see someone we find attractive or get sexually aroused. Pheromones are therefore an important key to human sexual attraction, although they are mostly undetectable at a conscious level, because they have powerful effects on our moods.

Japanese pillow books

Pillow books were a traditional gift exchanged between lovers; they take their name from the lacquered wooden pillows of Japan in which these conveniently small works or erotic instructions were traditionally kept. The first pillow book to bear the evocative title was written by a Japanese noblewoman early in the tenth and eleventh centuries, but erotic giftbooks have been enjoyed by lovers in China and India for many thousands of years.

Taoist sex

Sex puts a sparkle in the eye,
a glow to the cheeks
and makes the world seem like a better place.
Mantak Chia, Taoist Secrets of Love

Over two thousand years ago, Taoist physicians studying sex concluded that it is necessary to the physical, mental, and spiritual well-being of men and women. According to Taoist belief, energy and impetus are the source of a fulfilling existence. In the universe, humans are relatively small. In order to maintain a dynamic balance of health, we must be in accord with the source that is the immeasurable power of nature.

Taoism is not a cult, a religion, or a path to salvation; the Tao is the boundless force of nature, the path of the heart, or, put simply, "the way." The raw materials needed for the Tao can be found within ourselves at any given moment in our lives. The Taoists, being practical, proposed that we begin with the most accessible energy: the feeling of sexual attraction and the need to procreate. Unlike Tantra, Taoism never took on secret rituals and invocation of religious deities. Sex was more openly used in China as a medicinal form of healing and a natural way to spiritual balance.

There are two main goals for which the Tao technique of energy cultivation can be used:

- The first is to improve global happiness and to increase physical, emotional, and mental satisfaction. For example, the strengthening of love partnerships; alleviating sexual frustration, impotence, and premature ejaculation; relieving monotony with sex; and increasing longevity and good health.
- The second is to integrate sexual longing with one's spiritual belief or meditative practice. The Tao is a sex-positive approach that helps to better integrate sexuality with spiritual growth.

The beginning stages of Taoism, if you have a lover, are:

1. A man learns to sustain erection for as long as desired and regulates his ejaculation.
2. Both partners re-direct sexual energy through the body into the higher regions of the heart and brain.
3. The lovers exchange their super-charged energy with each other.

If you do not have a partner, you can follow what is called single cultivation where your sexual energy is used to restore the mind, body, and spirit in your daily life, so you can enjoy life without sexual frustration.

Tantric sex

Tantra is a cult of ecstasy, a personal religion based on the mystical experience of joy rather than established dogma. Sex is holy to a Tantric.

Kamala Devi, *The Eastern Way of Love*

Tantric sex is the Indian equivalent of Taoist sex. The major difference is that Tantra is seen to be a step on the road to spiritual enlightenment and mystical union, whereas practicing Taoist sex does not require a religious belief system but simply the development of willpower. The practice of Tantra, mind and body control reached from meditation and yoga, was born in India around 5000 BCE through the cult of the Hindu god Shiva and his consort the goddess Shakti. Shiva was worshipped as the embodiment of pure consciousness in its most ecstatic state, and Shakti as the embodiment of pure energy. The Hindus believed that through uniting spiritually and sexually with Shiva, Shakti gave form to his spirit and created the universe. Practitioners of Tantra, therefore, view the creation of the world as an erotic act of love.

The Sanskrit words for the genital organs are *lingam* for the man's and *yoni* for the woman's, and these organs, which to Westerners are associated with sex, birth, and nature, have in Indian culture a much more spiritual association. India's blatant enjoyment of sex has provided the world with the famous sex manual the *Kama Sutra* by the Indian nobleman and sage Vātsyāyana. *Kama Sutra* means "scripture of love." The *Kama Sutra* has many references to herbs and aromatics as an intrinsic part of the sexual act.

In Tantric practice, before sexual intercourse the woman is worshipped as the embodiment of the creative force Shakti. Her body parts are then anointed with different perfumes to honor her creative role and lift up her psyche so that she can manifest as a goddess. In the Rite of the Five Essentials, so called because all five senses would be aroused, the finest oil of jasmine is applied to the hands, oil of patchouli to the neck and cheeks, essence of amber or hina musk to the breasts, extract of spikenard to the hair, musk from the musk deer to the genitals, oil of sandalwood to the thighs, and essence of saffron to the feet. The man's body is also anointed with sandalwood oil.

What is the Tantra: a mystic cult, a magic ritual, a belief, a philosophy, or a spiritual practice? The Tantra may refer to the male and female sexual organs, as well as the sexual act itself, which is regarded as the symbol of sacred beliefs and divine bliss, and its means of attaining the ultimate goal through orgasm. It is difficult for many Westerners to understand its meaning and aims without oversimplifying and trivializing it. Centuries of religious and moral teachings, with their concepts of original sin and guilt, have clouded our minds so that it is difficult for us to accept that the sexual act can be a joy, a blessing, and a means to attain ultimate inspiration by precisely following a set liturgy and saying the appropriate mantras or prayers.

SMELL

All of us have our own unique smell. We cannot always detect it ourselves because our noses become satiated with one smell after a very short period of time, just as when we cannot smell perfume after half an hour or so. Your individual aroma is affected by your lifestyle, your diet, and your bathing habits. Desire, anger, and fear can also alter your smell as your body releases adrenaline.

Smell has very strong erotic connotations, and we can be attracted to or repelled by another person by the way he or she smells. Part of loving or desiring someone is loving their smell. Some North African tribes give so much credence to personal aroma that a wife can be instantly divorced if she does not smell right. Sexual excitement causes all sorts of exotic odors to emanate from the breath, the skin, and in particular the genitalia. In many successful relationships partners are able to recognize each other's smells, as the body's natural perfume is indeed a potent method of non-verbal communication. Smell has been linked with the "sixth sense," which is linked with our instinctive feelings about people. Honing in on these feelings can help us to read individuals better, which can be very useful within a sexual relationship.

Natural body perfumes can be enhanced by the subtlest of essential oils. Courtesans of medieval Europe used to wear a little of their vaginal secretions as perfume to attract others, dabbing it behind their ears and necks and on their chests.

Pubic hair

The ladies of the night of ancient Japan kept their pubic hair carefully plucked and clipped, and allegedly a knowledgeable man could "tell the degree of a woman's sexual skill by a mere glance at how she pruned her shrubbery."

Shaving your pubic hair is a bold step to take, and it itches when growing back. But trimming your pubic hair into a tidy groomed shape is very easy, not at all uncomfortable, and much more hygienic. And because hair retains fragrance after a trim, scented lotion can be applied so that a gentle fragrance will emanate from your pubic hair. Floral waters (hydrosols) of rose, ylang-ylang, neroli, or patchouli are popular scents.

A woman is like a fruit which will only yield its fragrance when rubbed by the hands. Take for example, the basil; unless it is warmed by the fingers it emits no perfume. And do you not know that unless amber be warmed and manipulated it retains its aroma within? It is the same with a woman; if you do not animate her with your frolics and kisses, with nibbling of her thighs and close embraces, you will not obtain what you desire.

Sheik Nefzawi, *The Perfumed Garden*

It's all in the mind

Sexual response begins in the mind; we have all heard or said, "I'm not in the mood." In his *Taoist Secrets of Love*, Mantak Chia says, "Sex really begins well in advance of the act, as the energies you accumulate then will express themselves when you go deep into sex; try to calm down any feeling of agitation or anger, as this more than anything else will block the flow of sexual energy." Closing down emotions to one's partner could easily have the effect of blocking the energy flow to other parts of the body, for example, the hormone system.

ORAL SEX

In India and China, oral sex has always been considered a normal part of the art of loving. In India, where the number of AIDS-infected individuals is severe, oral sex is recommended as a safer option, especially for young people. There is a profound skill in oral sex, and it is well worth learning. Both sexes should explore their own bodies to find out what is pleasurable, and foreplay with a partner is probably the most important part of any lovemaking. However, sexual hygiene is very important, and never more so when it comes to oral sex.

THE OLDEST APHRODISIACS

Several aphrodisiacs have been popular since the days of antiquity. The mandrake plant mentioned in the Bible's Old Testament is still used today. Mandrake is part of the potato family and has a large dark brown root and small red fruits. In mild doses its alkalis are soporific; in larger doses they can kill. In antiquity, there were magical rules for harvesting the plant. Pliny noted that the plant roots were in the form of human genitals, which explains the idea of the supposed aphrodisiac effect.

Ginseng was another old aphrodisiac made into tablets or put into wine and tea by modern sex-aid retailers. It is recommended to take a small glass of the wine before bed for its stimulatory effect.

THE MOST BIZARRE APHRODISIACS

Some of the most bizarre concoctions have been devised with the aim of restoring failing sexual powers. They can be plants with a resemblance to the human genital organs, but the most bizarre types of aphrodisiac are those involving an element of cannibalism. We know of the use of animal parts to increase human potency; a Chinese emperor, for example, kept a herd of deer so he could drink their blood to increase his virile power. But often it was thought desirable also to consume parts of men and women for this purpose. Menstrual blood, placenta, semen, and genitals have all been devoured to increase sexual prowess. Chinese eunuchs, seeking regeneration of their lost sexual organs, would eat the warm brains of newly decapitated criminals.

Some ancient recipes for aphrodisiacs are very peculiar and include body hairs. One recipe from the Middle Ages requires six pubic hairs and six hairs from the left armpit. The hairs would then be burned on a hot shovel and powdered. The resulting fine particles were then inserted into a piece of bread, which was dipped in soup and fed to a lover to rekindle his or her sexual interest.

Like body parts and certain foods, precious stones and pearls have been associated with the power to stimulate sexual desire, not only when presented as gifts, but also when consumed. Pulverized agate is supposedly especially effective. Cleopatra, successful seducer of Julius Caesar and Marc Antony, drank pearls dissolved in vinegar and honey. Precious gemstones have also been pulverized and used as makeup on the eyes. Ancient Persians used crushed pearls and rubies, gold dust, and ambergris to make pastilles that they ate as an aphrodisiac aid before sex.

In South America, some women have served coffee filtered through their underwear to the objects of their desire. A common aphrodisiac in ancient Rome was to cook a cow's vulva with other ingredients and serve to a prospective lover.

CHAPTER THREE

A–Z of Aphrodisiacs

A

ABSINTHE

(*Artemisia absinthium*)
Absinthe is a liqueur made in France manufactured from a bushy plant with silky stems and small yellow flowers, and is compounded of marjoram, oil of aniseed, and other aromatic oils. *Artemisia absinthium*, known as wormwood, was used to banish demons and was associated with the rites of St. John's Eve, when a crown of the plant was made to protect against evil spirits. Although absinthe has been considered a sexual stimulant, in large quantities it leads to impotence and insanity.
(Also see Wormwood)

ABUTA

(*Cissampelos pareira*)
Abuta is a beautiful woody vine, also known as "ice vine" or "velvet leaf," which climbs high over trees in the West Indies and South America. The dried root and bark are taken orally and contain a

variety of isoquinoline alkaloids that have great benefit for all with low sex drive, irregular menstruation, or childbirth problems. In Ecuador it is called the midwife herb and is reputed to reawaken an interest in sex after childbirth.

ACORUS CALAMUS

An aromatic herb that was called "sweet flag" in the Middle Ages. To ancient Romans, it was associated with many erotic practices and was known as the Venus plant.

AGATE

Like many other stones, precious and semiprecious, agate has a putative reputation for stimulating amorous activity. In the Middle Ages in particular, great trust was placed in the efficacy of such stones in the sense that they possessed talismanic virtues and were often used in love spells.

AGAVE

(*Agave americana*)
The many different species of agave are found in Central and South America. In Mexico they add the seeds of the thorn apple "datura" or the "ololiuqui vine" (*turbina corymbosa*) to the drink. Tequila is distilled from *Agave tequilana* other species are used in making a schnapps called mescal. In Oaxaca, a grub that lives in the agave stalk is often added to the beverage to increase sexual desire. It was widely used in pre-Columbian times as a medicine or tea and in religious ceremonies.

ALCOHOL

Alcohol with sugar was used to promote the amorous feelings of King Louis XIV. In some European countries, it was a folk custom to offer a bride and bridegroom cakes moistened with sugar or honey and alcohol. Francis I of France was also known for his cultivated taste and sexual prowess. He was notorious for the number of his lovers, but died of exhaustion from his excess of alcoholic aphrodisiacs.

Alstonia

(*Alstonia scholaris*)
This tree is also known as "dita," "bitter bark," "devil's tree," "pale mara," and "chatim." It grows in the rainforests of India, Ceylon, and Borneo. The bark was used as parchment by Asian scholars, leading to the name *scholaris*. The bark and seeds have also been used in Asian folk medicine for centuries. There are no proven aphrodisiac qualities, but myth says that it can prolong an erection and delay orgasm.

Ambergris

Ambergris is a waxy substance found in tropical seas, believed to be the secretion in the intestines of the sperm whale. In seventeenth-century France, courtiers and roués customarily nibbled chocolates covered with ambergris. Madame du Barry used ambergris as a perfume to retain the affection of Louis XV. According to one authority, three grains of ambergris are sufficient to produce lustful desires and to restore the fatigue of old age or overindulgence.

American ginseng

(*Panax quinquefolius*)
American ginseng is a robust, larger variety of the Manchurian ginseng root. It was used by the North American Indians as a medicine and for its aphrodisiac effects. The root was often used as a protective magical amulet or a love charm.

Angel water

Angel water was used by the Portuguese and was popular in the eighteenth century. Its ingredients are orange flower water, rose water, myrtle water, distilled spirit of musk, and spirit of ambergris. It is reputed to be a powerful aphrodisiacal aid when the genitals are bathed in the mixture.

Angel's trumpet

(*Brugmansia aurea*)

There are several species of angel's trumpet, or "tree datura," that grow in South America and other tropical areas. The angel's trumpet is a well-known Indian medicinal plant used by shamans as a hallucinogen. It is reputed to be a powerful aphrodisiac and stimulant.

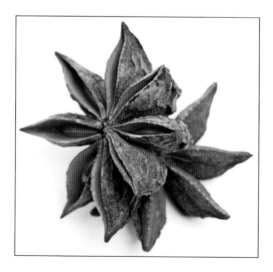

Aniseed

(*Pimpinella anisum*)

The anis bush grows in the Mediterranean region and has a long history of uses as a spice and medicinal fruit. Aniseed and star anise are both gently simulating aphrodisiacs that were used powdered and combined with honey to form a paste applied to the genitals in ancient India. Aniseed was also a central ingredient of the rich, spicy cake served at Roman weddings to encourage the sex drive of newlyweds.

ANNATTO

(*Bixa orellana*)
Annatto is a small tree native to South and Central America and the Caribbean. It has heart-shaped pods that contain seeds, of which a mature tree can produce six hundred pounds. In Colombia and Mexico, the leaves of the annatto tree are a valued aphrodisiac used to make a love tea. The pods are also decorated and used as talismans.

ANVALLI

Anvalli is a sexual stimulant mentioned in the Hindu erotic manual the *Ananga Ranga*. It consists of the outer shell of anvalli nuts, from which the juice is extracted. Dried in the sun, this juice is mixed with powder of the same nut and eaten with candied sugar, ghee or clarified butter, and honey.

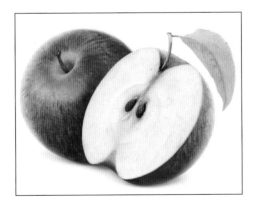

APPLES

Apples are a symbol of fertility that have always been associated with love, as they were sacred to Rhiannon, the Celtic goddess of love and marriage, as well as Viking and Greek love and fertility rituals.

In early British folk magic, a woman can enslave the man of her choice by sleeping with an apple next to her skin and then persuading him to eat it. Whether making the fruit into dumpling, tart, or turnover modified the magical effect is not recorded. In some ancient Scandinavian legends, the apple is described as the food of the gods. The belief was that the gods, grown old and decrepit, were rejuvenated by feasting on apples.

AQUAMARINE

An engraved aquamarine was used among Arabs as a love charm to secure conjugal fidelity. Aquamarine has been used for relieving stress and soothing nerves since at least 2000 BCE in Egypt and the East. The Romans believed it was lucky for lovers maintaining youth and health. Periapts, talismans, and various types of charms all play a prominent part in both European and Eastern erotology.

ARABIAN COFFEE

(*Coffea arabica*)

Coffee was formerly a sacred beverage; African Sufis drank it for its invigorating effect when meditating. The stimulation that coffee produces also helps with sexual dysfunction.

ARRIS

A Hindu technique is to take pieces of arris root, mix them with mango oil, place them in a hole in the trunk of the sisu tree, and leave them for six months. At the end of that time, an ointment is prepared that will effectively be applied to the penis. A woman will then go wild with desire for that man.

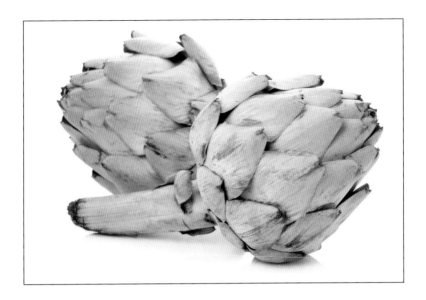

ARTICHOKE

(*Cynara scolymus*)
A bristly plant, sometimes known to North American Indians as "sun root," the artichoke was considered a powerful aphrodisiac, especially in France. Street vendors in Paris used to call:

Artichokes! Artichokes!
Heats the body and the spirit;
Heats the genitals.

Catherine de Medici was fond of artichokes. Eating artichokes may directly produce euphoria; indirectly, this sense of pleasant relaxation encourages intercourse.

ASAFOETIDA

(*Ferula assafoetida, Ferula narthex*)
Asafoetida is a plant with a turnip-like root, which contains a milky sap that thickens on contact with air into resinous granules that smell like garlic. It grows in India, Iran, and Afghanistan. The

granules are used in Ayurvedic and Tibetan medicine for their aphrodisiac value and are used in Asian cooking.

ASHWAGANDHA

(*Withania somnifera*)
Ashwagandha is a small evergreen shrub of the nightshade family native to India, the Mediterranean, and the Middle East. In Hindi or Sanskrit, the name means "sweat of a horse," as those who take it are said to attain the strength and sexual vitality of a horse. It has been widely used in Ayurvedic medicine for thousands of years as a *rasayan*, a rejuvenating or life-extending agent, and was among the most esteemed of Ayurvedic herbs. Ashwagandha is a renowned aphrodisiac that improves sexual performance and is sometimes used to treat impotence.

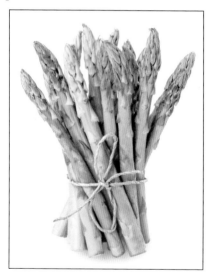

ASPARAGUS

(*Asparagus officinalis, Asparagus racemosus*)
The asparagus plant is a climber with tiny white flowers that is cultivated all over the world, but originates from India. The Egyptians,

Greeks, and Romans all valued asparagus as an aphrodisiac. According to an Arab manual, a daily dish of asparagus boiled and then fried in fat with egg yolks and a sprinkling of condiments will produce an erotic effect.

Its main use is as a galactagogue to increase milk secretion during lactation. It is also known to be useful for increasing the production of semen.

Ass

In Greek mythology the ass was the symbol of sexual potency. This animal was associated with satyrs and sileni. Pliny the Elder states that "to increase sexual potency, the right testes of an ass should be worn in a bracelet."

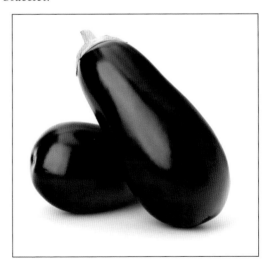

Aubergines

The aubergine, also known as eggplant or the apple of love, is regarded as an aphrodisiac in its native India. The *Kama Sutra* suggests rubbing your partner's body with aubergine juice to increase libido.

AVOCADO

(*Persea americana*)
The avocado tree originates from Central America and was cultivated by the Mayan Indians. It was used as a medicine for women's complaints and as a nutritious food. The oil was also prized in ritual as an anointing agent. The seeds and the flesh are considered an aphrodisiac to lend vigor and kindle sexual interest. The Aztecs called the avocado *abuáctl*, or testicle, a connection that seems to have impressed the Spanish conquistadores, who exported the fruit back to Spain as a food and sexual stimulant.

AYAHUASCA

(*Banisteriopsis caapi*)
The tree grows in tropical rain forests in the Amazon and is sacred to the Indians. It is also known as "caapi," "natema," and "yage." A psychedelic drug is made from the bark and shamans use it to go into healing trances. The drink is said to have an aphrodisiac effect and to produce feelings of euphoria. It works by stimulating the hormones that maintain the erection.

B

Ba ji tian

(*Morinda officinalis*)
Ba ji tian is a deciduous plant native to China. Its roots yield a pungent, sweet-tasting yellow dye. Ba ji tian is a popular sexual tonic that strengthens the erection and can help to overcome impotence and premature ejaculation. It is also used to help treat male and female infertility and hormonal problems.

Bananas

(*Musa acuminata Colla, Musa balbisiana Colla*)
Bananas are one of the few foods with real potential as an aphrodisiac not just for their phallic shape. The banana tree is actually an herb. Bananas contain an alkaloid (bufotenine) that acts on the brain to increase mood, self-confidence, and possibly sex drive. It is found in greatest quality just beneath the skin and is best obtained by cutting whole bananas lengthways and baking them with a little sugar or honey. The flesh should then be scraped away from the skin before eating.

Basil

(*Ocimum sanctum, Ocimum basilicum*)
There are a number of varieties of basil, all of which originate from South Asia. The basil plant has a reputation as a strong aphrodisiac in Mexico and Italy. In Italy, basil symbolizes love and is often used by girls as a love charm.

The tulasi plant, *Ocimum sanctum*, is one of the most holy plants of the Hindus. It is dedicated to the goddess Lakshmi and her husband Vishnu. The plant is said to provide abundant health and sexual vigor and is often planted in holy places and around altars.

BEANS

St. Jerome forbade nuns to partake of beans, ruled by Venus, because they were often considered an aphrodisiac food. In Italy, broad bean soup is often taken as an assumed aphrodisiac. Beans in general have long been believed to possess amatory virtue; being full of iron and protein, they do help strengthen the blood.

BEER

In England, common belief marks beer as a coital stimulus. Medical authority recommends that beer be taken with food, although too much beer will have the opposite effect. Beer is made with hops, which are full of the female hormone estrogen and thus may cause male beer drinkers to build up fat or develop breasts.

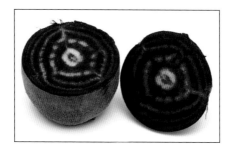

BEETS

White beets are described by Pliny the Elder, the Roman encyclopediast, as helping to promote amorous ability. In general beets, carrots, and turnips are all of aphrodisiac value and are also very good for your general health.

BETEL PALM

(*Areca catechu*)
Native to the tropical forests of Asia, the betel palm has small flowers and flamboyant orange or red fruit, the size of an egg, with hard

seeds. The nut is crushed and the seeds chewed to stimulate the body sexually and counteract intestinal parasites; it often leaves a stain on the mouth and can lead to the loosening of teeth. The seeds have been used in Ayurvedic medicine and in religious ceremonies as an offering to the gods.

BETEL PEPPER

(*Piper betle*)
The betel pepper is a climbing vine with dark green leaves from the tropical area of Southeast Asia. It is often used in an erotic curry and is very stimulating. Too much of the betel morsels will have an anti-aphrodisiac effect.

BHANG

Bhang is a Sanskrit term meaning "hemp." In India the leaves and seeds of hemp are chewed as a means of increasing sexual power. Frequently the seeds of hemp are mixed with musk, sugar, and ambergris as an aphrodisiac medication.
(Also see Hemp)

BIRD'S NEST SOUP

This is a Chinese dish said to be an extreme aphrodisiac, which has no flavor until it is highly spiced.

BIRDWORT

A shrub used in medieval times and by the Romans as an aphrodisiac.

BLACK COHOSH

(*Cimicifuga racemosa*)
Black cohosh, also known as "squaw root" or "black snakeroot," is an herbaceous perennial with creamy white flowers native to Canada and the eastern United States. The dried root of black cohosh is

mainly used as a relaxant, a uterine stimulant, and hormonal balancer by North American Indians.

BLACK MUSALI

(*Curculigo orchioides*)
A small perennial with an elongated tuberous root, stalk, and lateral roots, black musali grows wild in the Himalayas and India. It is an effective remedy for reproductive system problems. Legends of ancient times state that it is an herb that endows an individual with a great deal of strength and also has effective aphrodisiac qualities.

BLACK PEPPER

(*Piper nigrum Linn.*)
Pungent black pepper has a reputation for bringing spice to the bedroom as well as the palate. Pepper was so precious in ancient times that it was used as money to pay taxes, tributes, dowries, and rent. It was weighed like gold and used as a common medium of exchange. In 410 when Rome was captured, three thousand pounds of pepper were demanded as ransom.

BOIS BANDE

Loosely translated from its French origin as "potency wood," bois bande is a natural product administered in the West Indies by women that has the reputed virtue of an aphrodisiac. The ingredients contain a little strychnine and the bark of a tree that itself contains bucine. The bark of the tree of the same name is sometimes soaked in rum and drunk for sexual problems.

BLOOD

Human blood has often been used for anti-aphrodisiac purposes. Faustina, the wife of the emperor Antoninus Pius, fell in love with a gladiator. The magicians whom the emperor consulted advised that she drink her lover's blood to conceive a permanent hatred for him. In seventeenth-century Hungary, Countess Elizabeth Báthory was notorious for attempting to achieve rejuvenation by supposedly bathing in the blood of strangled virgins. She was caught and condemned to life imprisonment.

BONES

Camel bone is an aphrodisiac aid. Indian erotology suggests that camel bone be dipped in the juice of the *Eclipta prostrata* plant and burned. The black pigment from the ashes is placed in a box also made of camel bone and then applied with antimony to the eyelashes with a pencil of camel bone.

A Hindu erotic text suggests the stimulating and alluring effect of peacock or hyena bone covered with gold and tied to the right hand to induce sexual strength and power.

BRAINS

The brains of calf, sheep, and pig, young and served fresh, are reputedly erotic in their effects. As a side dish in Mediterranean countries, brains are a delicacy when properly prepared. The medieval philosopher and occultist Albertus Magnus wrote that brain could be used in formulas for love potions. He particularly recommended the brains of a partridge ground into a powder and swallowed in red wine.

BRASSICA ERUCA

The plant *Brassica eruca* was sown in the garden of medieval monasteries and taken daily by monks under the impression that it would cheer and rouse them from customary sluggishness. However, the continued use produced a very strong aphrodisiac effect.

BUTTERMILK

An anti-aphrodisiac, suggested in Hindu erotological literature as a way for women to negate amatory challenges, is to bathe in the buttermilk of a female buffalo. The milk is to be mixed with powders of the gopalika plant, the banu-padika plant, and yellow amaranth.

C

CABBAGE

Cabbage is used in many traditional aphrodisiac preparations. Cabbage is good for blood circulation due to its high iron level.

CACAO TREE

(*Theobroma cacao*)

The evergreen cacao tree grows in the Caribbean and in Central America. In the ancient Americas, cocoa was considered a food of the gods and was a popular aphrodisiac. Aztec prostitutes were paid in cocoa. Belief in the aphrodisiac value of chocolate prevailed for a long time. Seventeenth-century monks in France were forbidden to drink chocolate on account of its reputed aphrodisiac properties. The Sun King Louis XIV anticipated modern advertising by luring women to his bed with gifts of chocolate.

Eating chocolate can increase brain levels of several chemicals to produce a mild, confidence-instilling buzz. Chocolate also melts in the mouth at body temperature and so is very sensual to eat.

CAJUEIRO

(*Anacardium occidentale*)

Cajueiro, also known as the cashew, is an evergreen tree related to poison ivy and the mango, native to tropical America. The fruit of the cajueiro has a sweet flavor and is considered an aphrodisiac in Brazil. It is used together with catuaba and muira puama to treat impotence. The bark, said to be a contraceptive, is also used to make a treatment for vaginal discharge.

CAKES

In the Middle Ages, spiced cakes were often baked in a small oven over the naked body of a woman who wanted to retain the affections of her lover. This form of sympathetic magic was used to arouse desires in correspondence with the flaming heat of the oven. The baked creation would ultimately be offered to the object of the woman's love. Similar ceremonies are not unknown in other countries as well.

CALAMUS

(*Acorus calamus*)
This plant grows in the South Asian marshlands and North American plains. It has been used in medicine baths, teas, and incenses in many areas and is said to have a rejuvenating effect on the sexual life, best used in herbal baths to awaken sexual desire.

CAMPHOR

(*Cinnamomum camphora*)
Camphor is a concrete volatile oil obtained by distillation of water and the camphor tree wood. Mono-romated camphor is said to have an anaphrodisiac effect, but its great value is relief of colds, chills, inflammatory complaints, and irritation of the sexual organs. Sniff to lessen sexual desire and place beside the bed for this purpose.

CANNABIS INDICA

(*Cannabis sativa*)
Indian hemp is a drug that was used for centuries as an aphrodisiac. The plant grows in Central and West Asia and can be grown in many other parts of the world in the right conditions. One of the oldest archaeological relics in existence is a fragment of hemp cloth found at Çatal Hüyük that dates back to 8000 BCE.

In Istanbul, hemp seeds were customarily served at wedding dinners. During medieval times, cannabis was taken as a ceremonial drink in the temples of India to reach religious ecstasy. The use of cannabis can prolong and intensify the sexual experience, but prolonged use dulls the senses and can be an anti-aphrodisiac for some men.

Cantharides

(*Mylabris*)
Cantharides is a species of beetle found in southern Europe in which the principal irritant is a white powder called cantharidin. Cantharidin is toxic and may be fatal. It was widely used in the eighteenth century as a sexual stimulant and was inserted into biscuits, cakes, pastries, candies, and chocolates.

Caraway

(*Carum carvi*)
Caraway has a reputed aphrodisiac virtue; it is frequently mentioned in Eastern sex manuals and love or passion-inducing recipes. Several liqueurs are made with caraway, including Kümmel and some schnapps.

Cardamom

(*Elettaria cardamomum*)
Cardamom is an herbaceous plant found in the rain forests of Southeast Asia. When touched, it exudes a pleasant cinnamon scent. It is used to flavor food, especially rice, and beverages and has been known as an aphrodisiac since ancient times. A pounded mixture of cardamom spice seeds, ginger, and cinnamon sprinkled over boiled onions and green peas is considered in Arab countries to promote sexual vitality.

CARNATION

Magically, the flowers can be used in many rites of love and seduction. The petals are dried and scattered in potpourri or given in sachets to betrothed couples to keep their love life fresh and joyful. In incense or perfumes, carnations are used to increase personal magnetism and self-assurance. But white carnations can be made into an anti-aphrodisiac potion.

CARROT

(*Daucus carota*)
The ancient Greeks believed that all parts of the carrot were an aphrodisiac and ate the seeds, root, and foliage when preparing for an orgy. They were known as *philon*, meaning "loving," and were often given to potential sex partners to stimulate their passion. Among Arabs, carrots are eaten or stewed in milk sauce to help sexual activity.

CASTOR OIL

(*Ricinus communis*)
The castor oil plant is a native of India, where it bears several ancient Sanskrit names, the most ancient and most usual being *eranda*. Castor oil was once popular among North American Indians for erotic purposes; it was used as a base for mixing various herbs to prolong intercourse.

CATUABA

(*Erythroxylum catuaba, Juniperus brasiliensis, Anemopaegma mirandum*)
Catuaba is known as the "tree of togetherness" or the "tree of love" by the Tupí Indians in Brazil and is one of the most successful prosexual herbs available. The supplement is widely used to treat impotence and as an aid for fertility in older males. Catuaba tree bark contains aromatic resins and non-addictive alkaloids, catuabines, which are distantly related to cocaine. It acts as a sexual stimulant

and natural aphrodisiac, promoting erotic dreams and increased sexual energy in men and women.

CAVIAR

Caviar is in general considered to be a stimulant to sensual inclinations; it is invariably present at dinners and banquets that stress rich, erotic dishes accompanied by appropriate wines, resulting for the diners in a sense of widespread euphoria. Such a condition is highly conducive to amatory exercises, as European fiction illustrates so lavishly. The salty, musky aroma and pungent flavor of caviar is a renowned aphrodisiac that is said to remind lusty males of the female genitals. Caviar possibly contains steroidal compounds that might boost sex drive, but probably only in quantities that few today could afford.

CAYENNE

(*Capsicum frutescens*)
Cayenne, or chili pepper, is a perennial shrub native to Mexico and Central America, but now found through the tropics. Cayenne is widely known as a hot, spicy supplement that stimulates circulation to the hands, feet, and genitals and promotes sweating. It is sometimes used as a snuff and said to have aphrodisiac properties and help maintain an erection.

CEDAR

The tree is particularly sacred to the god Tammuz, the Assyrian vegetation god. Sacrificed each year by the goddess Ishtar, he thus alternates as god of the growing year and king of the underworld, where his consort is Ishtar's dark sister Ereshkigal. The oil and wood can be used in any incense or perfume dedicated to the horned one. As it is also a reputed aphrodisiac, it has very vigorous sexual properties and can be added to any seduction incense or pouch. Use with care.

CELERY

(Apium graveolens)
Celery, like the truffle, is said to contain an aphrodisiac substance similar to a pig pheromone that also has a pro-sexual action in humans. In eighteenth-century France, celery soup was a means of whetting the amorous appetite and was often included in love recipes.

CHAMELEON MILK

Chameleon milk was recommended as an erotic stimulant by Avicenna, a famous thirteenth-century Arab philosopher and physician. A noted libertine as well, he discussed erotic questions, sex procedures, and aphrodisiacs in his writing.

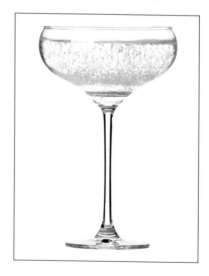

CHAMPAGNE

Long associated with erotic seduction, amatory relationships, and intimate dining. In general, wines have traditionally been of significant aid in amatory ventures. Champagne particularly excites the senses and is known as the wine of the bedroom; the feminine forms of champagne can even be made to blush.

CHARMS

Charms and potions of all kinds have historically been concocted for poisoning purposes or as love charms. Among ancient races, love charms were often associated with the technique known as sympathetic magic. The hoped-for result was similar to that of aphrodisiac stimulants. The ancients, such as the Greeks, felt that the human liver was the seat of all desires; hence it became a love fetish and aphrodisiac symbol. Among the strangest of charms is the udder of the hyena, tied on the left arm to entice the affection of any desired woman.

CHASTE TREE BERRY

(*Vitex agnus-castus*)

Agnus-castus also known as the chaste tree, is a deciduous, aromatic tree with palm-shaped leaves and small lilac flowers. It is native to the Mediterranean and West Asia and was traditionally used by monks to reduce sex drive, earning the name "monk's pepper tree." Chaste tree also has a reputation for boosting sex drive and fertility in women.

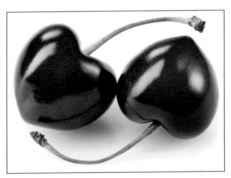

CHERRIES

(*Prunus serotina*)

Cherries, ruled by Venus, were considered stimulatory and often included in love cookery. Cherry bark has been used in magic to make your lover more passionate; wrap your lover's picture in red cloth along with the cherry bark to keep them keen.

CHILIES

Chilies can be added to food to arouse the interest of a reluctant lover. They are very powerful, but too much will have the opposite effect. Add them to a sachet or food to banish an unwanted lover.

CHILITO CACTUS

(*Epithelantha micromeris*)
The chilito is a round, thorny cactus that grows in Mexico and has red pepper-like fruits. The flesh of the fruit resembles chili peppers, thus the Mexican name chilito or "little chili." The Tarahumara people eat the fruit as a stimulant and an aphrodisiac; it is also reputed to repel evil forces.

CHOCOLATE

(*Theobroma cacao*)
Chocolate was sacred to Quetzalcoatl, the Aztec god of civilization and learning, and regarded as a powerful aphrodisiac in seventeenth-century Europe. The Sun King Louis XIV anticipated modern advertising by luring women to his bed with gifts of chocolate.

CHUCHUHUASI

(*Maytenus krukovii, Maytenus ebenifolia, Maytenus macrocarpa*)
Chuchuhuasi is prepared from the root bark of a large tree. When steeped in white rum for a week and mixed with honey, it is taken as one of the best-known jungle aphrodisiacs in Colombia and Peru. Chuchuhuasi is reputed to enhance virility, prolong erections, and cure male impotence.

Cinchona

A Peruvian bark that is used as a tonic, it has frequently been credited with the property of stimulating erotic expressions and prolonging erections.

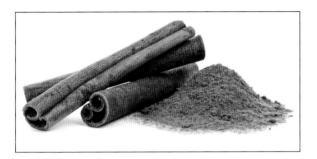

Cinnamon

(*Cinnamomum zeylanicum, Cinnamomum cassia*)
Cinnamon is the dried inner bark of an East India tree used as a spice with reputed erotic effect. Many centuries ago, a cinnamon liqueur was famous as an aphrodisiac at the courts of the Indian maharajas. The evergreen cinnamon grows in Southeast Asia. The young leaves are often bright red; in contrast, the flowers and fruits are small and inconspicuous. The bark is used in cooking as a spicy flavoring or made into an essential oil. The oil is used in the perfume industry; previously, it was rubbed on the genitals for erotic stimulation.

Civet

The civet mammal produced a musk that was widely used in perfume and said to be of aphrodisiac value. The nobility of the French royal court offered sweets perfumed with civet to desirable ladies. It is of interest to note that Daniel Defoe, author of *Robinson Crusoe*, was for a time owner of a civet farm.

Clary

(*Salvia sclarea*)
Clary is a plant closely related to sage. It has been used since ancient times as a spice and medicine. It was mentioned by the ancient Greek physician Dioscorides as having the ability to kindle sexual desire.

Cloves

(*Eugenia caryophyllata*)
The clove tree grows in tropical areas and has leathery leaves, tiny flowers, and long fruits. The clove has been used as an aphrodisiac for thousands of years, but overdoses can have very unpleasant side effects. Cloves are extremely useful in many rites of lust and seduction and can be used ether in incense, philters, or perfumes. A little of the essential oil added to any seduction oil encourages the opposite sex to desire physical contact.

Coca shrub

(*Erythroxylum coca*)
The coca shrub is indigenous to the South American Andes and has been cultivated for over three thousand years. Its leaves were used for oracular, medicinal, and religious purposes. The fresh leaves have long been chewed and made into a tea as a stimulant and as an aphrodisiac.

In ancient Indian cultures, the coca shrub was considered a gift from the gods and viewed as sacred. The coca shrub was also sacred to the Inca, who considered it the home of Mama Coca, a seductive, wonderful woman who could bless her devotees with her powers. Strict rules governed the use of coca leaves: they were offered to the gods, chewed in their honor, burned, or smoked. They were given to the populace during religious and state festivals as an aphrodisiac in religious and ritual acts. To ensure that Mama Coca was in a favorable mood, a collector was required to have slept with a woman before he went out to the coca harvest, and the leaves were then picked in her name.

The original Coca-Cola contained extract of coca leaves and cola nuts; it was very stimulating, was sold as a medicinal tonic, and certainly was an outstanding aphrodisiac. The success of the original beverage has not abated, even though the modern version contains neither cocaine nor the stimulating juice of the cola nut.

In 1859 Sigmund Freud published his experiences with coca leaves and cocaine in the *Centralblatt für die gesamte Therapie*. He also discussed its aphrodisiac effects, and cocaine became famous overnight. It very quickly became fashionable in circles fond of good living. Since its effect upon sexuality is so pronounced, its mere use became a disreputable erotic adventure; for many, however, what began as a stimulating recreational diversion became a fatal addiction.

All parts of the plant, but especially the fresh leaves, contain cocaine, the main active ingredient. This substance has a stimulating effect on the central nervous system and heightens the sensibilities. Coca has known effects upon the sphincter; it relieves pain and relaxes it.

Cocaine

Today cocaine is known as the magical white powder of the rich and super rich. Cocaine is correctly considered as an erotic drug or an aphrodisiac, as it enables greater control over orgasm. But cocaine is a very dangerous habit-forming drug whose use provokes sexual desire and excitement in both sexes, but particularly in women.

Coco de mer

(*Lodoicea maldivica*)
The coco de mer, or double coconut, appears wild only in the Seychelles archipelago. The resemblance to reproductive organs is

so vivid that rumor has it that the temple of Venus was carved in the wood. The natives believe that the palms unite as man and woman during stormy nights. Despite this, the coco de mer has no proven aphrodisiac properties.

COCONUT PALM

(*Cocos nucifera*)

Today the coconut palm grows all over the temperate world and is often cultivated in plantations and gardens. All parts of the plant can be utilized; the roots are made into traditional remedies, the flower stem is tapped to obtain palm wine, and the nut is eaten or used for its oil. Palm wine is said to be an energizer and aphrodisiac, and coconut milk mixed with thorn apple seeds and honey is a great tonic. Palm wine can also be distilled into powerful schnapps known as arak.

COLLYRIUM

Collyrium is a Latin term meaning "eye salve." These salves were used by the Romans and the Hindus and were reputed to have a stimulating effect on sexual relationships. In addition, collyrium was endowed with traditional magical properties as a love charm.

CORIANDER

(*Coriandrum sativum*)

This annual herb was introduced by the Romans, who adapted its use from the Greeks, to the Egyptians and Africans. Coriander seeds are mentioned in the *Tales from the Arabian Nights* and are still prized by Arabs as a famous aphrodisiac. To the ancient Chinese, coriander seeds were believed to confer immortality and possess magical regenerative powers. This is probably linked to its powers as a love potion. When the old herbals talk of herbs as a "rejuvenator," they mean the restoration of youthful sexual vigor rather than the smoothing of wrinkles and the restoring of youth.

COTTON

(*Gossypium herbaceum*)
The seeds of the cotton plant contain valuable oil. In China, the roots of the cotton plant were used to inhibit the production of semen. In the Ayurvedic system, the root cortex of the cotton plant is considered a tonic and rejuvenator.

COUNTRY MALLOW

(*Sida cordifolia*)
Country mallow is a plant with strong roots and sturdy stature grown in India. It has been found useful for problems with the reproductive system and is used in Ayurvedic medicine for sexual dysfunction, such as impotence and low sperm count.

COW WHEAT

(*Melampyrum pratense*)
Cow wheat is a tall plant with yellow flowers, used to feed cows. But Pliny the Elder, Roman encyclopediast, and Dioscorides, physician, said that it inflames desire and amatory passions.

CRESS

(*Apium nodiflorum*)
Cress is most often used in salads and as a dressing for food. It is said to be an aphrodisiac if eaten raw or boiled or drunk as a juice. The plant was cultivated in Italy and the East for its sexual value. Ovid, Martial, and Columella, all Roman poets, testify to its erotic power.

CROCODILE

Crocodile teeth attached to the right arm will act as an aphrodisiac, states Pliny the Elder in his *Historia Naturalis*. Crocodile tail is also a sexual delicacy, as is crocodile excrement, according to the Roman poet Horace.

CUBEB

(*Piper cubeba*)

The cubeb is a berry similar to a grain of pepper with a very pungent flavor. It is used in cookery and in medicine. A drink made from cubeb pepper is described as a strong aphrodisiac in many Arabic manuals. Chewing cubeb pepper also produces similar results, as does powdered cubeb mixed with honey or wine. In China, an infusion of cubeb pepper leaves is prepared as a highly stimulating aphrodisiac.

CUCUMBER

(*Cucumis sativus*)

Cucumber probably gains its reputation as an aphrodisiac due to its suggestive shape and length. In fact, the fruit of the cucumber hinders lust when eaten, but the seeds are said to promote fertility and are good for the urinary system.

CUP OF GOLD

(*Solandra brevicalyx*)

Cup of gold is a climbing plant that grows in the Americas. It has long yellow funnel-shaped flowers. Cup of gold was cultivated in Mexico as an ornamental, magical, and medicinal plant. The women of the Lacandon Maya used the flowers to perfume their clothes and attract men. Other members of the tribe used them to make an aphrodisiac drink. The Aztecs also mixed the leaves with cocoa to blend an erotic love drink.

D

Damiana

(*Turnera diffusa aphrodisiaca*)

A small shrub with aromatic leaves native to Central America, Mexico, Namibia, and the Caribbean. It can be smoked and brewed as a tea or alcohol. Its volatile, aromatic oils and beta-sitosterol stimulate the sexual organs and gently irritate the urogenital tract to produce a local stimulant effect with tingling and throbbing sensations. Its alkaloids may also boost circulation and increase the sensitivity of nerve endings in the genital area. Damiana also increases circulation to the penis so that erections are firmer and last longer, thus increasing sexual desire. It is one of the very few substances that can be considered a true aphrodisiac, as it works directly on the genital organs as a tonic stimulant.

It is a powerful aphrodisiac and is very potent and vigorous in love rites, particularly helpful to one seeking a magical partner. It can be toxic and cause liver damage, so it may be safer to use it in incense to attract or heighten sexual abandon.

The Maya considered asthma a disease that evil winds carried into the body. Not only does it cause shortness of breath and possibly depression, it can also make a person impotent and destroy all sexual desire. With the aid of damiana, however, a person afflicted with asthma can regain joy of life and sexual desire. Physicians from other cultures have also seen a connection between asthma and impotence or sexual desire.

Darnel

(*Lolium temulentum*)

Bearded darnel is sometimes known as "cheat" or "tare." It is used by doctors to treat dizziness, insomnia, blood congestion, stomach problems, and skin problems. Darnel is a grass that, if sprinkled with frankincense, myrrh, and barley meal, is reputed to be a sexual aid for women. This herb is poisonous in large quantities and is not to be used without medical direction.

DATE PALM

(Phoenix dactylifera)
The date palm was probably cultivated in Mesopotamia some eight thousand years ago. Preserved dates are believed by many gourmets to have erotic stimulus. They are rich in vitamins and have more calorific value than steak; they have been used in love feasts for thousands of years.

DILL

(Anethum graveolens)
Dill was often used in the East as an ingredient in aphrodisiac meals and in magic. The seeds are used in love philters and potions, particularly in mulled wine as an aphrodisiac. For this purpose, you may also add a drop or two of the essential oil or an infusion of seeds to your bath to make you irresistible to the opposite sex. The oil also makes a good addition to any massage oil. Many Roman herbals single out dill as one of the most potent of all aphrodisiac plants.

DONG QUAI

(Angelica sinensis, Angelica polymorpha)
Dong quai, sometimes spelled "dang gui" or "tang kuei," is native to China and Japan, where it grows deep in mountain ravines, meadows, and riverbanks. It may help to boost sexuality in women with low sex drive and is linked with menopausal symptoms, heavy periods, and menstrual cramps. It is said to increase blood circulation to the pelvis and regulate the menstrual cycle.

DRUMSTICK TREE

(*Albizia lebbeck*)

The drumstick tree can grow up to sixty feet high and is planted on roadsides for shade in India. A juice is made from drumstick flowers, which are used in recipes for many medicines, including asthma, and a treatment for insect bites. It is also regarded as a promoter of virility.

DURIAN

(*Durio zibethinus*)

The durian tree produces hedgehog-sized brown fruits, which are known variously as "stink fruits," "stink nuts," and "tree cheese." The fruit has a rotten smell and is not allowed to be carried on public transportation in many countries. The ripe fruit has a reputation as an especially powerful aphrodisiac throughout Southeast Asia and is often used in folk medicine. It is so highly prized as an aphrodisiac that owners frequently sleep under the trees at harvest time to protect their crop.

E

Echinacea

(*Echinacea angustifolia, Echinacea purpurea*)
Echinacea, also known as purple coneflower, is an herb indigenous to North America. Native Americans claim that it enhances resistance to infections such as the common cold. It reputedly can also help with loss of libido. The hydrosol can be used as a sexual wash and has immunity-boosting properties.

Eggs

Eggs, especially free-range eggs, contain steroidal substances that seem to enhance libido. An egg yolk in a small glass of cognac, drunk every morning, has been popular as an aphrodisiac in France. In Morocco, love philters are composed of egg yolk and bedbugs. Many Eastern aphrodisiac dishes frequently contain eggs as an ingredient.

Elecampane

(Inula helenium)
Elecampane is mixed with vervain and mistletoe to make a love powder. It was recommended by Nicholas Culpeper as an aid in regulating women's problems and for digestive and urinary problems.

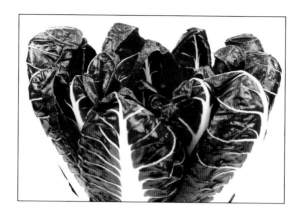

ENDIVE

(*Cichorium endivia*)
Endive, like a number of similar plants, is both edible and reputed to have aphrodisiac properties.

EPENA

(*Anadenanthera peregrina*)
Epena is a mimosa-like tree from the South American rain forests. The natives of the Orinoco basin used the seeds to go into psychedelic trances. It is also used by shamans to contact spirit guides for healing. It has a reputed aphrodisiac power and can increase sexual vigor.

ERYNGO

(*Eryngium maritimum*)
Also known as "sea holly" and "sea hulver." The testicle-shaped root of this plant was extraordinarily popular in Regency Britain as an aphrodisiac. In Shakespeare's *The Merry Wives of Windsor* Falstaff mentions it: "Hail kissing-comfits, and snow eryngoes." The root has been candied to strengthen the genitals and give potency; in this form the Arabs knew it as an invigorating sexual stimulant.

F

FALSE UNICORN

(*Chamaelirium luteum, Helonias dioica*)
False unicorn is a perennial herb from North America, which is also known as "blazing star" and "fairy wind." It is chewed by Native American women to help prevent miscarriage and is also said to have aphrodisiac properties.

FENNEL

(*Foeniculum vulgare*)
A fragrant plant used in sauces and believed to inspire sexual provocations. Fennel soup is a dish used to stimulate desire in some Mediterranean regions. Fennel has great magical affinity with the serpent deities and can thus be very helpful in the gentle release of kundalini energy. It can also be used in small doses in love potions and, if eaten with eel, was reputed to promote strong lustful feelings.

Eating fennel is said to stimulate the genitals and arouse desire. Even the dew gathered from the leaves of fennel was believed to have magical powers, including strengthening both physical sight and magical clairvoyance.

FIGS

The fig is considered sensual and erotic for its apparent resemblance to the female genitals. In some cultures, figs are eaten at weddings and thrown at newlyweds in the place of rice.

The fig tree figures in the founding of great cultures and religions. Romulus and Remus, the founders of Rome, were suckled by a she-wolf under a fig tree, which was later revered as a sacred tree. While sitting under a fig tree, Siddhartha Gautama had the revelation that formed the foundations of Buddhism.

Figs have been prized for both medicinal and dietary value. Mithridates, the Greek king of Pontus, heralded figs as an antidote for all ailments and instructed his physicians to consider its uses as a medicine. The early Greeks so highly valued figs that it was considered an honor to bestow the foliage and fruit. In the original Olympic Games, winning athletes were crowned with fig wreaths and given figs to eat.

FISH

Many aphrodisiac recipes from various cultures and periods of history contain seafood. Fish is considered a powerful and unfailing erotic aid particularly on account of its phosphates and iodine.

According to Apuleius, fish was used as love charms. A fish bone is often included in magical sachets and lucky amulets. In Egypt, the aphrodisiac virtues of fish were so generally recognized that priests were forbidden to eat fish when they had to remain celibate.

FLEAWORT

(Psyllium)
Fleawort is well known as a traditional aphrodisiac. The sap of this plant, according to Pliny the Elder, was an effective means of securing the birth of a male child. The would-be parents drank the sap three times daily while fasting for forty days.

FO-TI

(Polygonum multiforme)
Fo-ti, also known as *he shou wu*, is a perennial climber native to central and southern China. It is one of the oldest Chinese tonic herbs used to prevent aging. Fo-ti is famous for its rejuvenating and revitalizing properties. It is widely used by millions of men and

women in the East as a general restorative and to promote fertility and sex drive.

Fo-ti-tieng

(*Hydrocotyle asiatica minor*)
This Asian perennial plant has purple flowers and flat, rounded leaves. It is reputed that the leaves, taken daily, prolong life and act as an aphrodisiac. Fo-ti-tieng was used widely in Sri Lanka and China.

Frog

According to the medical writer Alexander Benedictus, dried frog powder induced a disgust of sexual activities, but frog bones were used among the Romans as aphrodisiacs.

G

Gall

The gall of a jackal was used as an aphrodisiac by Arabs. It is specifically recommended as an ointment for this purpose by Sheik Nefzawi, author of *The Perfumed Garden*.

Garlic

(*Allium sativum*)

Eating garlic can improve feelings of well-being and sex drive. It is reputed by many erotologists to have aphrodisiac value. The Romans consecrated it to Ceres, the goddess of fertility, and made a love cocktail from pressed garlic juice and coriander. It is now medically proved that garlic can help with erectile dysfunction, as it has a chemical constitution that helps with lowering cholesterol and in de-furring blood vessels leading to the penis.

Ghee

In Hindu custom, ghee, or clarified butter, is considered an aphrodisiac. An ancient Hindu manual on erotica suggests boiled ghee, drunk in springtime mornings, as a health-strengthening beverage.

Ginger

(*Zingiber officinale Roscoe*)

Ginger is a perennial, tropical plant native to the jungles of Southeast Asia. Ginger is one of the oldest medicinal spices and aphrodisiacs known. It was taken regularly by Confucius, who helped to make it popular in China for medical and erotic purposes. Ginger is an energizing spice that can increase blood circulation and liven up your sex drive.

GINKGO

(*Ginkgo biloba*)

The Ginkgo biloba, or maidenhair tree, is one of the oldest known plants, often described as a living fossil. It boosts blood circulation to the brain, hands, feet, and genitals by stopping platelets from clumping together. Research shows that it can improve blood flow to the penis and help maintain an erection.

Ginkgo is one of the most popular health supplements in Europe today, where it helps to improve memory and concentration and is used in treating dementia. It was considered sacred in China and Japan and is planted on Taoist, Buddhist, and Shinto temple grounds. Since ancient times, the sacred tree has had great importance as a healing plant in Chinese medicine.

GINSENG

(*Panax ginseng*)

Ginseng is a perennial plant native to northeastern China, eastern Russia, and North Korea; it is now rare in the wild. Ginseng is a true pro-sexual supplement and adaptogen, prized as a sexual enhancer and fertility aid. It can be grated and eaten in soups and salads or dried and powered for use in teas and tablets. The Chinese have revered this plant for thousands of years. Like mandrake, the most potent ginseng roots are said to be shaped like the human body.

GOAT

The goat was associated with the Greek gods Aphrodite, Dionysus, and Pan on account of its amorous tendencies. The Greek physician Dioscorides extolled the virtues of goat's milk and recommended cabbage steeped in goat's milk as an arouser agent. The *sicinnis* is a Greek erotic dance that represented the jumping of goats and was associated with the sensual ways of satyrs. In the West Indies, goat curry with spices is known to be an aphrodisiac.

Goji berries

Goji berries come from the Himalayas and are said to contain five hundred times more vitamin C than oranges do. Studies show that they fight fatigue, lift libido, aid digestion, and even help eliminate cellulite.

Goose

The goose has often traditionally been seen as a symbol of potency. Goose tongues were recommended by the Roman poet Ovid for their aphrodisiac qualities. Goose grease is often used in herbal ointments and salves.

Gotu kola

(*Centella asiatica, Hydrocotyle asiatica*)
Gotu kola is an herbaceous perennial plant native to India, China, Indonesia, Australia, and the South Pacific. It is reputed to increase longevity and is also referred to as the fountain of youth. Legend claims that gotu kola was one of the herbs used by Li Ching-Yun, a Chinese herbalist who reputedly lived to the age of 256. It is one of the most important Ayurvedic herbs and boosts energy and sex drive.

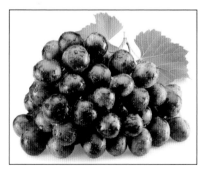

Grapes

(*Vitis vinifera*)
The grapevine is one of the world's oldest cultivated plants, consumed as a fruit, raisins, or wine. Its original home was in Asia

Minor, but today it grows throughout the world. Grape juice is a reputed aphrodisiac, as are wine and alcohol, which lower the inhibitions but dampen the sexual urge if overly imbibed.

Guarana

(*Papaver somniferum*)
The guarana liana is a climbing shrub with divided compound leaves and yellow flowers that grows in the rain forests of the Amazon. Its chestnut-like fruits have been called the fruits of youth by the locals. For centuries, the Indians of the Amazon have collected the seeds for a very stimulating drink. It is also used as an appetite suppressant and is often found in slimming preparations, and is used for psychic protection.

Guayaca wood

(*Guayacum sanctum*)
The guayaca is an evergreen tree that grows in Central America. Its wood is known as "wood of life." The Indians of Central America use the wood to manufacture hunting bows because of its hardness, which is supposed to transfer to the penis.

H

Hashish

(*Cannabis indica*)
The Indian hemp plant is chewed, smoked, and drunk. The term "assassin" is derived from the Arabic *hashishin*, "hemp eaters," that is, drug addicts. Hashish has a demoralizing effect, replacing inhibitions with emotional excitement. The sense of moral responsibility is lost, together with all willpower. The aphrodisiac effect stems from the creation of such excitement and abandonment and loss of restraint and moral sensibilities.

In the case of marijuana, as inhibitions are removed, the smoker becomes highly suggestible toward sexual expression, but long-term use will cause moroseness, lethargy, and sexual ineptitude.

Hemlock

(*Conium maculatum*)
Hemlock was much used in ancient times, but is considered too dangerous today. The Greek biographer Plutarch describes the medicinal properties of the herb and its poisonous effect. In the eighteenth century, hemlock was used for treating cancer, syphilis, and ulcers.

Hemp

(*Cannabis sativa*)
Hemp, one of humanity's oldest cultivated plants, was used as a food and source of fiber as well as to dull pain and prolong active life. It is considered an active aphrodisiac, as it eases pain, lowers inhibitions, and relaxes the body to enrich the erotic experience.

Henbane

(Hyoscyamus niger)

A drug is obtained from the flowering plant henbane, which grows in England and Europe. The plant has large, sea green leaves and cream-colored flowers streaked with purple. It is eaten by hogs and pigs, but is deadly poisonous to humans. In rural European areas, it was smoked like tobacco, but produced convulsions and hallucinations. Witches were said to have used the plant for madness-inducing love potions. It is also an anti-aphrodisiac and is fatal in large doses.

Henna

The pulverized leaves and twigs of henna are used as a hair dye in many European countries and as skin decoration in India and the East. Among Arabs it is believed that henna rubbed on the fingers, skull, and feet produces an aphrodisiac reaction. Indian women's hands and feet are decorated with henna on their wedding day for this reason.

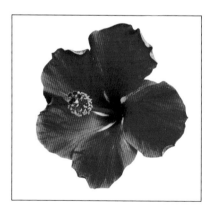

Hibiscus

Hibiscus originates from India, but now grows in gardens all over the world. Hibiscus flowers can be used with love incenses or carried as a love potion. In Ayurvedic literature, hibiscus flowers are known to have anti-fertility effects and are used for birth control and as a treatment for menorrhagia. It is also used to cure impotence and promote virility.

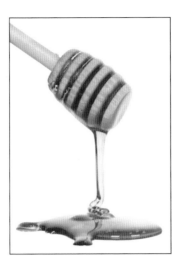

Honey

According to the Roman poet Ovid, author of the *Ars Amatoria*, honey is a great aphrodisiac. In ancient India, honey was widely used in growth poultices applied to the penis and mixed with crocodile dung, olive oil, and lemon juice for a contraceptive barrier by women. Honey can also be used as a lubricant and a delicious introduction to the pleasures of oral sex.

In Arabia, honey and yogurt were often used on genitalia as a prelude to oral sex. As a contraceptive aid, bee pollen is said to increase the biological value of the egg and sexual stamina as well as restore and rejuvenate natural hormonal substances.

Horny goat weed

(*Epimedium sagittatum*)
Horny goat weed grows wild in China and is traditionally known as "lusty goat herb" and "yin yang huo." It is popular in the East

but not so often used in the West. Horny goat weed is used to treat impotence and lowered fertility in men. It is said to increase blood flow to the penis and boost waning libidos in both men and women. The exact way it works is still unclear, but it is believed to increase testosterone and levels of the brain chemicals required for sexual arousal.

HORSERADISH

(*Armoracia rusticana*)
Used in Europe as a condiment, horseradish is reputed to have a stimulating sexual value. The root is similar in appearance to a penis and is said to help with sexual exhaustion and general fatigue.

HORSETAIL

(*Equisetum myriochaetum*)
Horsetail is indigenous to Central American rain forests. Fresh segments of the stalk are made into teas for treating many ailments; the Lacandon people make one specifically for aphrodisiac purposes, which is said to improve hardness and stamina of the male sexual organ.

HYPERICUM

(*Hypericum perforatum*)
Hypericum is a perennial shrub found in many parts of the world, especially Europe and the United States. It is also called St. John's Wort, from the knights of St. John of Jerusalem who used it as a salve during the Crusades.

Hypericum has bright yellow flowers and small oval leaves. It has been used for over two thousand years to treat depression, low self-esteem, and sleep problems. It is said to boost the level of feel-good hormones in the body and to aid in low sex drive.

I

IBOGA

(*Tabernanthe iboga*)

This bush grows in the Congo and West African rain forests; the shrub has white flowers with pink spots and a berry with seeds. It has been used as a fetish plant and is well known by West African cults and sacred societies as a sacramental plant. The root is also considered to be one of the strongest African aphrodisiacs and is often combined with yohimbe bark in aphrodisiac potions.

INDIAN ALOE

(*Aloe indica*)

Aloe has large fleshy leaves and is native to eastern and southern Africa. Used as a promoter of virility and menstruation, the fresh juice is a tonic to help soothe penile inflammation and skin complaints.

INDIAN KUDZU

(*Ipomoea digitata*)

Indian kudzu is a vine with a woody stem, pink flowers, and hairy brown seeds. It grows in the Himalayas and Nepal and is used as a promoter of semen, an aphrodisiac, and a general tonic.

IPORURO

(*Alchornea floribunda*)

Iporuro is a shrub that is native to the Amazon; its bark is harvested in the dry season when it contains a number of active ingredients, including yohimbine, a powerful treatment for impotence. The Ticuna Indians use iporuro to both increase the fertility of females and to treat male erectile dysfunction. It is taken fairly widely by older men as a general tonic and aphrodisiac.

J

Jangida

(*Withania somnifera*)
This bushy plant grows in South Asia and has small bell-shaped flowers and red fruit. The plant was used in Vedic magical rites and Ayurvedic medicine. Chinese medicine used it as a curative and as an aphrodisiac. Love drinks made from the fruit are said to promote sexual vitality and arousal in any person.

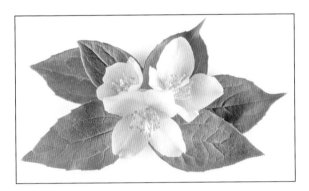

Jasmine

(*Jasminum*)
A flower with a beautiful fragrance, jasmine is known to Hindu poets as "Moonlight of the Grove." It is used mainly in the form of an exotic essential oil, which can be very expensive if pure due to requiring around eight thousand handpicked flowers to make a single drop.

Juniper

(*Juniperus communis*)
Juniper is a shrub that produces fleshy purple berries with a pungent taste. It yields oil that is used medicinally and in massage.

Juniper is also credited with the virtue of maintaining an erection and giving youthful ardor to tired men. In North America, Native American tribes made a tea from juniper berries, which they drank as a contraceptive.

JUSTICIA

(*Justicia pectoralis*)

This plant grows in the open clearings all over Central America and in the Caribbean, where it is considered an aphrodisiac. The entire plant is dried in the sun and made into a powder, which is taken like snuff or smoked with cannabis.

K

KAVA

(*Piper methysticum*)

Kava, sometimes referred to as "kava-kava," is a Polynesian perennial plant related to the pepper found in the South Sea Islands. It has heart-shaped leaves and short spikes that are covered with flowers. Its botanical name *Piper methysticum* literally means "intoxicating pepper" because it was used for thousands of years to brew an intoxicating alcoholic drink called Kava. This drink is said to be a natural tranquilizer that helps with insomnia and sometimes causes vivid erotic dreams. Kava has been used in rituals of Tantric yoga and is said to initiate blissful feelings, resulting in it being used as a supplement for depression.

KORIBO

(*Tanaecium nocturnum*)

This liana thrives in the tropical and coastal zones of South America and Central America. The delicate flowers are closed during the day, only opening at dusk to give out an intoxicating aroma similar to that of almonds. The Choco Indians use the root cortex to make an aphrodisiac tea.

KUILI

According to the Hindu manual *Ananga Ranga*, a drink containing kuili powder, cucumber, asparagus, milk, and other ingredients is highly strengthening to the sexual urge.

L

Land caltrops

(*Tribulus terrestris*)
Land caltrops, also known as puncture vine, is a high-altitude perennial trailing plant that grows wild in Africa. Known to be an excellent aphrodisiac for the elderly and over-tired, it is also used for urinary disorders, incontinence, and impotence.

Laurel leaves

(*Laurus nobilis Linnaeus*)
Laurel leaves were widely used to promote amatory exercise and in love charms in the East. According to Pliny the Elder, the tradition of placing wreaths upon the brows of victors began with Livia Drusilla, the wife of Caesar Augustus. Legend says a hen holding a sprig of laurel was dropped in Livia's lap by an eagle. Afterward the emperor, when going out in triumph, held a laurel branch from the original tree in his hand and wore a wreath of its foliage on his head, and subsequently every one of the ruling Caesars did the same.

Lavender

(*Lavandula angustifolia*)
Small doses of lavender are said to cause sexual excitation, and a few flowers in tobacco induce a dream-like state. Lavender essential oil is a good addition to any massage mix. Romans used it for its beautiful fragrance, antiseptic quality, and protective associations, the plant being sacred to the goddess Vesta. Sex-starved Empress Josephine served a chocolate and lavender concoction to her husband Napoleon when her thoughts and attentions turned to sexual delights.

LEEKS

(*Allium*)
Like its close relations garlic and onions, leeks have a long reputation as a powerful aphrodisiac.

LENTILS

Lentils were widely used in ancient Greece and were believed to stimulate sexual desire. In the sixth century, chickpeas were believed to be an aphrodisiac, while curiously enough, lentils were considered to have the opposite effect. This was probably the reason why the lentil was included in monastery diets on meatless days.

LING ZHI

(*Ganoderma lucidum*)
Ling zhi has been called the "mushroom of immortality" and the "phantom mushroom" due to its rarity. There are many legends concerning its magical powers. The mushroom became a symbol of long health and a sexually fulfilled life to Taoists. Elixirs of immortality and powerful aphrodisiacs were brewed with it.

LICORICE

(*Glycyrrhiza glabra*)
Licorice is an herbaceous plant whose roots are valued in confectionary and medicine. Licorice is used for a tonic for the adrenal glands and digestive and intestinal problems. It has been added to recipes for many aphrodisiacs and incenses, as it is reputed to incite strong sexual passion. It is also an aromatic ingredient in any smoking mixture. The pleasant quality of true licorice led to it being incorporated into many traditional Chinese remedies, where it was credited with harmonizing the body's response.

Liver

Dried liver was used by the Romans as an ingredient in love potions. Horace, the Roman poet, mentions this as a popular aphrodisiac.

Lizard

Lizards were favored in many Arab countries for their aphrodisiac qualities. Aelius, an Alexandrian physician of the second century, recommended lizard flesh to ensure virility. The flesh is powdered and drunk with sweet wine, providing erotic stimulus. Lizards were brought by Egyptians to Cairo and shipped to the Mediterranean ports, particularly Marseilles and Venice, where they were much sought after as aphrodisiacs.

Lotus

(*Nelumbo nucifera*)
The lotus flower grows like a water lily in still waters, ponds, and gardens. It is considered to be the birthplace of gods and is viewed as a symbol of enlightenment, eternal life, and spiritual development. It is said that lotus flowers sprang up from the ground in the footsteps of the Buddha. It has long been used as a medicine, healing food, and aphrodisiac.

Lovage

(*Levisticum officinale*)
Lovage originates in Southwest Asia, but is now grown in many gardens. Both the herbage and the root have been considered aphrodisiacs. The fresh root is used to prepare a love drink. The plant is considered the "rod of love," a symbol with an unambiguous male component.

LYCOPODIUM

(*Lycopodium clavatum*)

Lycopodium is a plant with a claw-like root, once believed to have aphrodisiac properties. It is often used in homeopathic medicine as a mood regulator.

M

Maca

(*Lepidium meyenii*)
Maca is a root vegetable related to the potato that is grown in the Central Peruvian Andes. Its tubers contain a number of steroid glycosides with estrogen-like effects. Dried and powdered maca is used to increase energy and stamina and can aid female fertility and male impotence.

According to Peruvian history, during the height of their empire, Incan warriors would devour maca before entering into battle. The maca would imbue them with a fierce strength and made the Inca into a daunting adversary; but after entering the conquered city, the soldiers were forbidden from eating it to protect the native women from the powerful sexual impulses of the invading force. The dried root was also used as currency by the Inca. They considered maca a gift from the gods, along with potatoes and corn, and it was used by shamans in medicine rites.

Maca is also used for stress and depression, but too much of the herb acts as a laxative, probably because of its high fiber content.

Maerua arenaria

(*Hybanthus enneaspermus*)
Maerua arenaria is an herb native to India, which is widely used to promote desire and sexual vigor.

Mandrake

(*Atropa mandragora, Mandragora officinarum*)
This plant is sometimes called mandragora and belongs to the potato family. It has dark leaves, purple flowers, and a tomato-like fruit that is the size of a large plum and emits a peculiar odor. It

is indigenous to the Mediterranean area and Palestine. The mandrake was often used in ancient times to stupefy criminals who had been sentenced to death. Shakespeare referred to it as a soporific in *Othello* and *Antony and Cleopatra*. It was also administered to surgical patients by the ancient Greeks and in the Middle Ages.

The mandrake is one of the plants and herbs that resemble the human genitalia and thus has been associated with aphrodisiac qualities, which modern science has since confirmed. In Roman times it was often used in love charms and philters. Columella, a first-century poet, called mandrake "maddening" because it was believed to form a component in love potions that were intended to drive victims mad with desire. Young men of Athens carried pieces of mandrake with them as love charms as late as the nineteenth century.

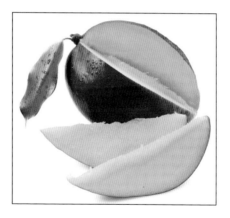

MANGO

The name "mango" is derived from the Tamil word "mangkay" and has been known as the food of the gods for as long as four thousand years. The mango tree plays a sanctified role in India as a symbol of love and possibly wish-granting. Mango leaves are used at weddings to ensure couples conceive plenty of children. The fruit is featured prominently in Hindu erotology, believed to boost sex drive and prolong lovemaking.

Marigold

Bathing in marigold infusion is said to infuse your aura with the power to attract the opposite sex. Marigold is good for the heart, raises spirits, and increases sexual stamina.

Marjoram

(*Origanum majorana*)
Marjoram is an aromatic herb often used in cookery for flavoring foods. Among the Romans, marjoram was known to have an aphrodisiac value. Sweet marjoram essential oil can be used in massage oil mixes to enhance sleep and relaxation.

Marrow

According to tradition, bone marrow is a source of vitality. A marrow paste was a common concoction for heightening the sexual appetite. The Roman poet Horace refers to dried marrow as a reliable aphrodisiac.

Matico

(*Piper angustifolium*)
This pepper plant grows in the tropical regions of the Americas. The Indians of Central and South America used them as a spice. In pre-Columbian times, the leaves were used to treat wounds, but the fruit and leaves were used as an aphrodisiac.

Matwu

(*Cacalia cordifolia*)
A shrub native to the Americas, it has heart-shaped leaves and yellow flowers. It belongs to the so-called "false peyote" plants that are used in ritual in place of peyote and is used to treat fatigue and sterility.

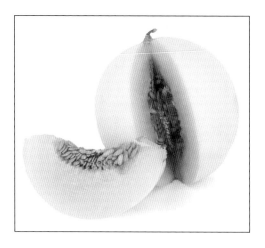

Melons

In ancient Persia, melons were considered an aphrodisiac and eaten regularly to stimulate the appetite for both food and love. Melon is still commonly served as a starter for seduction meals in many cultures.

Mescaline

(*Prosopis*)

Mescaline is a substance derived from the tufts of the peyote cactus that grows wild in Central America, Mexico, and Texas. This cactus appears as a cluster of small button-like growths, the main root being underground. The small growths, when dried, are known as peyotl or mescal buttons. They are bitter and leathery in texture.

In Mexican folklore, the use of this drug is well documented. The cactus was called "flesh of the gods" and was an object of worship among native Indian priests. The Spaniards who invaded Mexico called the cactus "devil flesh." In parts of South America, the mescal button was harvested in a religious ceremony. In some locations, stone statues are fashioned in the shape of the buttons and worshipped.

Over time, the use of peyotl was extended throughout South America, Mexico, and Central and North America. At the end of the nineteenth century, scientists began to examine the properties of the cactus and its effects on the mind and body. Some test subjects disclosed remarkable visions and hallucinations after taking the mescal infusion. Mescaline is a very dangerous drug and should never be taken without medical supervision.

MILK

Among Arabs, washing the genitals in ass's milk was considered a means of stimulation. Poppaea, the wife of the Roman emperor Nero, and Cleopatra are said to have bathed in ass's milk for beautifying purposes. In India, brides and grooms are sometimes given warm milk on their wedding nights to give them stamina.

MILK THISTLE

(*Silybum marianum, Carduus marianus*)
Milk thistle is a thorny, weed-like plant with purple flowers native to the Mediterranean. Milk thistle seeds contain a powerful mixture of the antioxidant bioflavonoid known as silymarin. Silymarin can help improve liver function, which may in turn raise testosterone levels and help to improve low sex drive.

MINERAL WATERS

Bathing in specified mineral waters has for many centuries been considered an aphrodisiac tool. The procedure was well known to the ancient Romans, who constantly practiced it in resorts throughout the Roman Empire. In Arabic texts dedicated to erotic advice, bathing in them is recommended to increase sexual vigor.

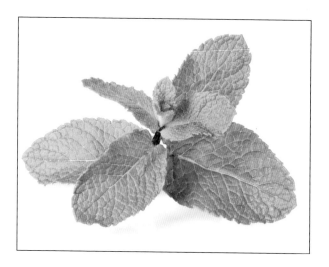

MINT

According to the classical erotologist Mattioli, mint is an herb that is effective in strengthening male vigor and is reputed to have aphrodisiac properties.

MISTLETOE

(Viscum album)

Mistletoe is sacred to the gods Hermes, Cernunnos, Balder, and Freya. From the earliest times, mistletoe has been one of the most magical, mysterious, and sacred plants of European folklore. It was considered a giver of life and fertility, a protector against poison, and an aphrodisiac. Mistletoe was long regarded as both a sexual symbol and the "soul" of the oak. It was gathered at both midsummer and winter solstices, and the custom of using mistletoe to decorate houses at Christmas is a survival of the Druid and other pre-Christian traditions. Mistletoe is still ceremonially plucked on Midsummer's Eve in a number of Celtic and Scandinavian countries.

The tradition of kissing under the mistletoe is first linked with the Greek festival of Saturnalia and later with primitive marriage rites. Mistletoe was believed to have the power of bestowing fertility, and the dung from which the mistletoe was thought to arise was also said to have "life-giving" power. In Scandinavia, mistletoe was considered a plant of peace, under which enemies could declare a truce for warring spouses to kiss and make up.

In certain parts of England, mistletoe is burned on the twelfth night of Christmas lest all the boys and girls who have kissed under it never marry. And for those who wish to observe the correct etiquette, a man should pluck a berry every time he kisses a woman under the mistletoe, and when the last berry is gone, there should be no more kissing!

MOLY

(*Allium*)
Moly is a legendary herb with white flowers and black roots that is credited with magical qualities. In *The Odyssey*, Hermes gives the herb to Ulysses to protect him against the guile of Circe. It is credited with everything from being an aphrodisiac to preventing the Black Death during the Middle Ages.

MOON FOAM

The stuff of legend historically prized by Morocco's witches, moon foam is a legendary powerful substance that captures the essence of the new moon. It can allegedly enforce a lover's fidelity, cure or prevent impotence, repair male or female fertility, and instill mad, crazy passion to whoever uses it. There is little doubt that the moon affects the female reproductive system; the best time to conceive is said to be on the waxing moon. Passions seem to run higher during a full moon as well.

MORNING GLORY

(*Ipomoea violacea*)

Morning glory flowers are native to the Americas and thrive in the clear areas of the Central American rain forests. The seeds were used in pre-Columbian times for medicinal and ritual purposes. An ideal aphrodisiac for women, it was consumed at religious festivals. The seeds, which Indian healers believe to be the home of a god, contain lysergic acid that helps geological and urinary conditions. However, overuse of these plants can cause miscarriage and psychedelic effects.

MOTHERWORT

(*Leonurus cardiaca*)

Motherwort probably derives its name from its use as a sedative infusion, taken to ease the pain of childbirth and menstrual problems and to prevent miscarriages. Some people recommend this plant to increase male virility or help with any sexual problems that are attributed to anxiety or stress.

Because of its affinity with Venus, motherwort can also be used in many love spells, but it is quite an unpleasant-tasting herb, so keep it to a minimum in potions or philters. If you add the herb or infusion to your bath water, it is said to draw lovers to you like moths to a flame.

MUGWORT

(*Artemisia vulgaris*)

Mugwort is a slightly different species than wormwood, but of the same genus and oils. This waterside plant was used in the East as an aphrodisiac. It is also recommended by Culpeper to induce menstruation and for treatment during labor and after pregnancy. Use in a bath or as an ointment. The name Artemisia is from the goddess Artemis, who inspired the plant's genus name.

MUIRA PUAMA

(Ptychopetalum olacoides, Liriosma ovata)

Muira puama is a small tree with white flowers that smell like jasmine that is found in the Brazilian rain forest. It is widely used by natives of the Amazon and Orinoco river basins to enhance sexual desire and combat impotence. It has an extremely hard timber, the wood and bark of which are boiled to make an alcoholic drink. Muira puama is also known as "potency wood" or "tree of virility" in Brazil and is used as a tonic. Taken as a tea, it is used to treat sexual impediments, improve potency, and prevent baldness.

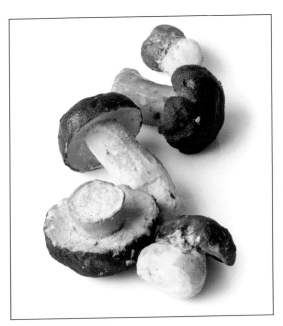

MUSHROOMS

Raw mushrooms, like truffles, have an odor reminiscent of sex and were widely regarded as aphrodisiacs by the ancient Romans and Greeks and Arabs. There are numerous varieties of mushroom that have toxic properties, which were mentioned liberally by medicinal texts as far back as the Middle Ages.

MUSK

(*Moschus moschiferus*)

Musk is a brown, bitter, and volatile substance, extracted from a gland near the genitals of the musk deer and of a species of goat indigenous to Tartary. In Persia and Tibet, musk is used in food for its amatory properties.

The smell of musk is associated with the ideal woman, according to the *Kama Sutra*. Arab writers commented on the effectiveness of perfuming oneself with musk as an aid of enhancement before sexual activity. Musk could also be taken internally to stimulate the male genitals, according to old medical records of the eighteenth century. Musk was in the past often used in perfumes and preparations, but its use is now prohibited in most parts of the world. Musk is a potent stimulant and aphrodisiac.

MUSK ROSE

(*Rosa moschata*)

Musk rose is a very special perfume, as it acts as a combination of the love powers of Venus and the lustful energies of the Horned God. This perfume is also helpful to those involved in Tantric magic or in rituals of sex or seduction. Try using just a little to perfume the belly, as this is reputed to inflame the senses of your partner.

For those who find the energies of pure musk too powerful or wish to temper lustful longings with love and friendship, musk rose is an ideal substitution, being derived from plant material and not animal.

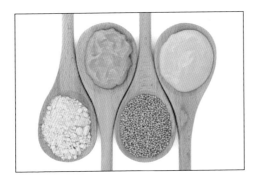

MUSTARD

(*Brassica nigra*)

Since ancient times, both mustard seeds and plant have been attributed with virility-promoting effects. For this reason monks were forbidden to use mustard. It is often documented that hot mustard baths are recommended to assist and enhance women's libido.

MYRRH

(*Commiphora myrrha*)

A composite of eggs boiled with myrrh, pepper, and cinnamon, taken on several consecutive days, is recommended by many Arabs for strengthening amorous vigor. The gum is especially prized in the East and used as a medicinal aid for various illnesses as well as an erotic stimulant. The essential oil of myrrh can also be used in massage mixes.

MYRTLE

In the Middle Ages, pulverized myrtle leaves were applied to the body as a sexual stimulant. Myrtle has long been known as an ingredient in love spells and love baths. When the goddess Aphrodite arose from the sea where she was formed, she plucked sprigs from a myrtle bush to cover herself. It is said the myrtle lips and fruit are shaped like the labia majora and labia minora respectively.

N

Nail clippings

According to the ancient Romans, nail clippings, sometimes with hair, were used in magic rites for aphrodisiac purposes or to attract or control a prospective partner.

Nepenthes

Nepenthes is a drug or potion mentioned by Homer as having the effect of banishing sorrow or mental inhibitions. It has been variously identified with opium, hashish, and *panax chironium* by Theophrastus, a third-century BCE Greek philosopher who wrote some volumes of beneficial plants. He also asserts that this drug was administered as an aphrodisiac infused in wine.

Nettle

(*Urtica dioica*)
The stinging nettle is a perennial plant found worldwide, though few people realize its medicinal effects, especially on the urinary system. Nettle extracts seem to increase testosterone and sex drive. In many cultures, flagellation with nettles was exercised upon the buttocks and adjacent parts to have a powerful effect upon the genitals.

The Romans frequently used urtication, beating with nettles, to arouse the sexual appetite and treat skin disease. Nettle tea is also good for the heart, skin, blood, and bones because it is high in minerals.

Niando

(*Alchornea floribunda*)
This bushy plant is native to Africa and has been used since ancient times in magic and religious ceremonies. It induces hallucinations

and can, if taken as a beverage, invoke blissful feelings; it is known as a powerful aphrodisiac.

NUTMEG

(Myristica fragrans)

Nutmeg is an aromatic seed of a tree native to Indonesia that is used to spice food and is highly prized in the East as an aphrodisiac. Nutmeg contains an amphetamine-like chemical that is harmless in small quantities. If, however, grated nutmeg is mashed with avocado flesh and chilled overnight, a chemical reaction occurs that is said to produce a pro-sexual effect in men. The nut and the fruit are diuretic, galactagogues, and stimulants.

NUX VOMICA

(Strychnos nux-vomica)

This wild tree grows in Asia and has broad leaves, crown-like umbels, and orange fruit. When dried, the seeds are also known as "poison nuts" or "crows' eyes." Nux vomica is a drug that may have stimulating aphrodisiac effects and is effective in cases of impotence, but also causes hallucinations and should never be used without medical supervision.

O

OATS

(*Avena sativa*)

Oats are a nutritious aphrodisiac that may be taken as porridge or in supplement form. Its reputation as a pro-sexual herb may account for the popular saying "sowing one's wild oats." Oats are a wild grass that may have originated in the Middle East or the Mediterranean basin. Some of the earliest evidence of their use is found in cave drawings in northern Europe that date to 1000 BCE.

ONIONS

Like their relation garlic, onions are reputed to be a powerful aphrodisiac to the point that celibate Egyptian priests were forbidden to eat them. Ovid advised that eating onions stirred the passions. Onion soup is recommended in France as a restorative after a fatiguing first wedding night.

OPIUM

(*Papaver somniferum*)

Opium is extracted from the poppy, which was cultivated as a garden flower for thousands of years. In ancient Sumeria, opium was known as the "plant of joy." In the Middle Ages, it was used for medicinal and soporific purposes and also for eating and smoking. Later it acquired an acknowledged aphrodisiac significance. English medicine received its first experimentation with opium in the Middle Ages from Venice via Germany. It journeyed from Asia Minor in the fifteenth century, traveled across India to Macedonia and Persia, and began to be cultivated in the eighteenth century.

Theophrastus, Pliny the Elder, and Roman biographer Cornelius Nepos refer to opium medicinally. Opium removes inhibitions and enhances excitement, but does not physically act as an aphrodisiac. Opium and its derivatives, including morphine, are all habit-forming drugs, dangerous if not fatal.

ORCHIS

(*Orchis morio*)

Orchis morio is a plant of the Satyrion species grown on the mountains near Istanbul. Its root was used in ancient times as the basis of a powerful aphrodisiac called Satyrion. The orchis are small orchids that grow in meadows, harvested during magical rituals and prepared with a number of other ingredients as beverages or spiced foods. Used in Ayurvedic medicine and by health practitioners in ancient Greece as a tonic and sexual stimulant, it was viewed as a wondrous agent of love.

P

Parsley

(*Apium petroselinum*)
This is used for garnishing foods and is traditionally considered an effective aid in aphrodisiac meals. Parsley has always been a favorite garden plant and was considered a symbol of rebirth in ancient times. The root was used in sachets to attract love and induce erotic ecstasy.

Passionflower fruit

(*Passiflora incarnata*)
The passion vine's flower structure is said to symbolize the crucifixion of Jesus: the inner corona of filaments represent the crown of thorns and the styles depict the cross and nails. The passion fruit is commonly regarded as an aphrodisiac, but passionflower tea is better used as a cure for insomnia and excited nerves. Passionflowers are often used in love magic and love charms.

Pepper

(*Piper nigrum*)
Genuine or black pepper is a climbing vine found only in the tropics. Both Asian and European folk medicinal traditions consider white, black, and red pepper superior aphrodisiacs.

Pfaffia

(*Pfaffia paniculata, Pfaffia stenophylla*)
Pfaffia, also known as "suma," "Brazilian ginseng," and "Brazilian carrots," is a ground-covering vine found in Brazilian forests. It is regarded as a remedy for all ills. It has been used as a female aphrodisiac and to treat male impotence for at least three hundred years.

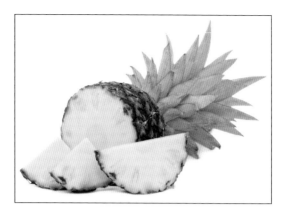

PINEAPPLE

(*Ananas comosus*)

The pineapple is one of many fruits to be considered an aphrodisiac. Now grown worldwide but originally from South America, the pineapple has for centuries been used in medicine. It is an excellent diuretic and is very good for the metabolism.

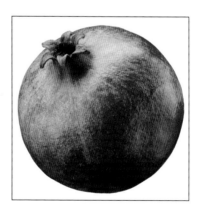

POMEGRANATE

(*Punica granatum*)

The pomegranate is a small tree originally from Southwest Asia, but now grown all over the Mediterranean. It is often called the "apple of love," as it was venerated as a symbol of the goddesses Astarte and Aphrodite. The pomegranate is believed by some to be the fruit, rather than the apple, that tempted Eve in the Garden of Eden. The *Kama Sutra* recommends splitting the blushing golden globe in two and sharing it for a night of incomparable passion and boosted fertility.

POPPY

(*Papaver somniferum*)
The opium poppy is now found worldwide and has many different-ent colored flowers. It has become enormously important because of opium, which is obtained from the thick milky sap extracted from the seed pod. This was used as a medicine, inebriate, and aphrodisiac.

PRICKLY ASH BARK

(*Zanthoxylum americanum*)
Prickly ash bark is traditionally used to increase circulation, especially in the lower half of the body, and to help with sexual potency.

PUFFBALL

(*Elaphomyces cervinus*)
The puffball is a fungus that gets its name from the grayish-violet powder it produces. It is also known as "hart's truffle." Since ancient times it has been considered an aphrodisiac for both humans and animals, but it is very toxic and can have dangerous side effects.

Q

QAT

(*Catha edulis*)

The qat bush is grown wild in Northeast Africa and Arabia. It was well known to the ancient Egyptians, who considered it a divine plant. Qat is used fresh; it can be chewed, made into sweets with honey, or mixed into beverages like coffee. The dried leaves can be smoked alone or blended with hashish. Its effects are said to include mystical insights and trances as well as sexual feelings.

QUEBRACHO

(*Aspidosperma quebracho-blanco*)

This yellow-blossomed tree grows in the tropic grasslands. Its bark is used in medicine and as an aphrodisiac. It is made into a beer that has contraceptive and abortive properties.

R

Rauvolfia

(*Rauvolfia serpentina*)

Rauvolfia, also known as "reserpine," is a drug used to reduce high blood pressure. In Sanskrit, the plant is known as *sarpagandha*, which means "insanity cure." The drug is extracted from the dried root of the plant and has been used in India for thousands of years as a medication for headaches and circulation problems. It also produces erotic dreams with various aphrodisiac effects.

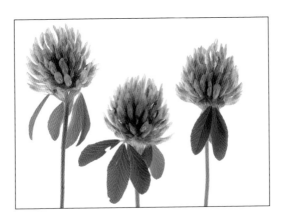

Red clover

(*Trifolium pratense*)

Red clover, also known as "cow clover," "beebread," "purple clover," and "trefoil," is native to Europe and Asia. It is used to balance estrogen levels and treat menstrual problems. It can greatly benefit women with low sex drives.

Rhodiola rosea

Rhodiola rosea grows in Siberia and is also known as "golden root." It has been used to enhance sexual stamina and treat stress and impotence. *Rhodiola rosea* became such a legendary invigorating agent that Chinese emperors sent expeditions to Siberia to gather the root, which can be taken in teas and supplements. In Siberia, it is traditional for married couples to receive a bouquet of *Rhodiola rosea* roots on their wedding night.

Rocket

(Brassica eruca)
Rocket is a species of cabbage that grows in the Mediterranean and is often used in salads. The plant has been especially celebrated by the ancient poets, including Ovid, Marital, Horace, and Columella, for restoring vigor to the sexual organs.

Rose

(Rosa spp.)
Rose oil is used in aromatherapy for its calming and relaxing properties. It is also well known as an aphrodisiac, especially in combination with sandalwood oil in massage. Magically, the rose can be used in many ways, especially for love.

The ancient Greeks said that the rose was formed from the body of a dead nymph that Chloris, goddess of flowers, found in the forest. When Chloris called on the other gods to aid in creating the flower, Aphrodite gave the rose beauty surpassing all others, the three Graces gave youthful blossoming, brilliance, and joy, and Dionysus gave it an intoxicating nectar and perfume. Finally Chloris crowned the flower with dewdrops and declared it queen of the flowers.

Victorian women used to pick petals from the most fragrant roses and cover them with egg whites beaten in water. Then they dusted them in superfine sugar to crystallize them and dried the petals on parchment. These were then given as love gifts to their suitors.

Rosemary

(*Rosmarinus officinalis*)

Rosemary is an aromatic shrub indigenous to southern Europe. The leaves are used medicinally, in perfume, and in cookery. It was reputed as an aphrodisiacal stimulant by the Romans. The best aphrodisiac effect results from taking a rosemary bath to stimulate the brain, circulation, and skin and increase sensibilities.

S

Safflower

(*Carthamus*)
Safflower is a thistle-like plant that was highly recommended as a sexual stimulant in the fourth century. Safflower can be beneficial for women with hormonal problems or those approaching menopause, when sexual desire can diminish.

Saffron

(*Crocus sativus*)
Saffron, the dried pistils of a crocus, is considered a powerful aphrodisiac in Egypt, Greece, Spain, India, and China. It is traditionally taken to maintain sexual performance in males and in cases of general debility. Saffron was used by the ancient Phoenicians as a spice to flavor the moon-shaped cakes eaten in honor of Ashtoreth, the goddess of fertility.

Sage

(*Salvia officinalis*)
Sage is a well-known culinary herb traditionally associated with a long, healthy life. Sage is used to help reduce excessive sweating and is a popular herbal remedy for treating hot flashes and night sweats. Clary sage is a euphoriant and antidepressant; some find it an aphrodisiac. Sage is reputed to have an incredible effect on women and is used in love philters to make the drinker irresistible to the woman he or she desires.

SALEP

Salep is a jelly-like preparation made from the dried root of the *Orchis morio*. It is used in the Middle East as a drug and food. In Turkey, Iran, and Syria, salep is popular as a sexual restorative.

SAN PEDRO CACTUS

(*Trichocereus pachanoi*)
This cactus grows in South America and can reach up to twenty feet tall. It has been used ritually and medicinally since ancient times. Fresh slices of the cactus are used to brew a drink that is used in shamanism to produce visions and healing trances. It is also well known as an aphrodisiac.

SANDALWOOD

(*Santalum album*)
Sandalwood is a tree with scented leaves that is often used in aromatherapy or in aphrodisiac recipes. It is a sacred oil used in many Indian love rituals.

SARSAPARILLA

(*Smilax officinalis*)
Sarsaparilla, also popularly known as "smilax," belongs to a group of climbing perennial vines that are armed with prickly spines and are found in tropical and subtropical areas around the world. The dried, thick rhizomes and slender roots are widely used in herbal medicine. Sarsaparilla has been used as a male pro-sexual herb since ancient times; it was introduced to Europe in the fourteenth century by the Spanish.

It is used to increase low sex drive in men and to help overcome impotence and infertility because it aids testosterone production. It can be used in lower doses in women to boost low sex drive and help with menopausal symptoms.

Sauerkraut

According to researchers in Pittsburgh, sauerkraut has a definite sexual effect on men, supposedly due to its high content of vitamin C and lactic acid.

Savory

(*Satureja montana*)
The Romans cultivated this pungent herb purely for its supposed aphrodisiac qualities. It was usually taken with honey, which could be mixed with wine. This herb was also advocated by the poet Ovid as a sexual stimulant. Regular use boosts immune function and, if used with cinnamon and oregano hydrolates, can enhance libido.

Saw palmetto

(*Sabal serrulata, Serenoa repens*)
The saw palmetto is a small palm tree native to North America and the West Indies. It has long been used as a male tonic, sexual rejuvenator, aphrodisiac, and to stimulate breast enlargement in women.

Schisandra

(*Schisandra chinensis*)
Schisandra, also known as "magnolia vine," is an aromatic woody vine native to northeastern China. It is a popular Chinese tonic herb commonly used by Taoist women to enhance their sexual energy. Like ginseng, schisandra has powerful adaptogen properties and appears to be a true pro-sexual herb. It helps the body adapt and cope with stress and is well known as a sexual tonic that reputedly increases secretion of sexual fluids in men and women.

Scotch pine

(*Pinus sylvestris*)
Used as a hydrosol, scotch pine is one of the best general tonics and an effective immune system stimulant. The essential oil has a mild hormone-like effect on the endocrine system. Scotch pine improves physical and mental strength and should be used in baths and saunas.

Sea bean

(*Canavalia maritima*)
Sea bean is a squat bush found in South America and Africa with red flowers and bean-like fruits. The beans have been used in Africa for thousands of years as an aphrodisiac and have been found in prehistoric graves. They are also smoked as a marijuana substitute together with the dried leaves. In Peru, the plant has been used in rural magic and sex rites.

Sensitive plant

(*Mimosa pudica*)
The sensitive plant responds to touch and is found in many places in India, Africa, America, and Brazil. It is widely used for urinary complaints and bleeding disorders such as menorrhagia. The seeds help to increase the production of semen and provide vigor and vitality for men.

Siberian ginseng

(*Eleutherococcus senticosus*)
Siberian ginseng is a deciduous, hardy shrub native to eastern Russia, China, Korea, and Japan. It was first discussed as a valuable medicine over two thousand years ago in the herbal thesis *Divine Husbandman's Classic of the Materia Medica*, which refers to the root

of Siberian ginseng as a panacea for maintaining health. For this reason it was regarded as a treasure by the ancient sages.

Siberian ginseng is widely believed to increase one's zest for life and is noted for its aphrodisiac properties. It has estrogen-like activity and has been shown to relieve hot flashes, vaginal dryness, night sweats, and anxiety. It is also said to improve fertility by enhancing overall vitality and regulating sex hormones for women.

SKINK

(*Scincus officinalis*)
The skink is a small lizard indigenous to Arabia and North Africa. It has been prized as a medicine and is treated throughout Arabia as a potent aphrodisiac when fried in oil.

SNAKE

During the Renaissance, philters in France called *goblet d'amour* often contained the heart and tongue of a viper, and the blood and hair of a redheaded woman. Snake meat is prized in the East for its invigorating properties.

SPANISH FLY

Spanish fly has long been known to increase sexual desire, arouse the female libido, and even improve the female orgasm. The Spanish fly, which is actually the emerald-green blister beetle, is found in the southern parts of Europe. The crushed and dried body of the beetle was used as a diuretic and a very potent aphrodisiac. It works by irritating the urogenital tract and producing itch in the sensitive membranes, allegedly increasing the desire for sex.

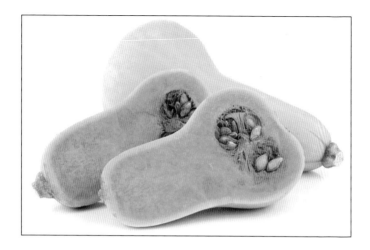

Squash

(*Cucurbita pepo*)
The squash has large, round fruits and yellow flowers. The seeds are eaten and used medicinally and were long considered an aphrodisiac. The Ayurvedic and Tantric systems have long valued the seed, as they belong to the class of *vajikarana* aphrodisiacs that are consumed during Tantric rituals of love.

Stinkhorn

(*Phallus impudicus*)
This fungus is often found in the forests of Germany and has become well known because of its shape and smell. It has been called "witch's egg" or "devil's egg" and is an ancient aphrodisiac.

Stramonium

(*Datura stramonium*)
This plant is sometimes called "thorn apple." It is a strong narcotic drug largely used in the East. Stramonium seed, mixed in wine, produces a sexual stimulus, but can be fatal in large doses.

Strawberry

Strawberries are known as the "fruit of Venus," the Roman goddess of love. They are regarded as an aphrodisiac, especially when combined with champagne. The oil can be used in perfumes, sachets, and baths to attract love or to awaken passion.

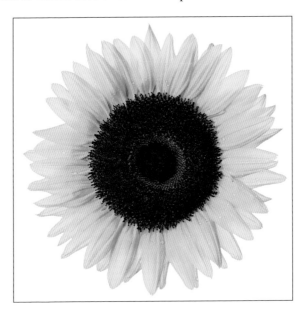

Sunflower

(*Helianthus annuus*)
The sunflower has been cultivated for over three thousand years in Mexico. It has long been used as a remedy and food, and the oil is now used all over the world. The Mayans made an extract of the petals, which they drank as an aphrodisiac.

Sweet flag

(*Acorus calamus*)
The sweet flag is grown all over the temperate world in marshes and near streams and ponds. It has been used for over two thousand years

by the Chinese, the Mosuo sorcerers of Yunnan, and in Ayurvedic medicine. The Cree Indians of Alberta would chew a piece of root to overcome fatigue, produce hallucinations, and enhance sexual stamina.

SWEET POTATO

(*Ipomoea batatas*)
The delicious sweet potato forms long, turnip-like roots and has been cultivated in South America for many thousands of years. It is eaten boiled, baked, or fried and has a reputation as a female sexual stimulant. As a remedy it is useful for women in menopause or with menstrual problems, as it contains trace amounts of estrogen.

SYRIAN RUE

(*Peganum harmala*)
Syrian rue, also known as "harmel weed," is a bushy shrub found in deserts or desert-like regions. Since ancient times, the plant was used for religious and magical ceremonies. Shamans inhale the smoke in order to enter ecstatic states. The aphrodisiac effect of the plant, in particular the seeds, is well documented.

T

TEA SHRUB

(*Thea sinensis*)
The tea shrub originated in China, but is now cultivated throughout Asia. It has been used as a tonic drink for more than three thousand years. Tea was popular among the Taoists as a stimulant and an aid for contemplation and meditation. It was also used as an aphrodisiac, usually in conjunction with other substances such as ginseng or opium.

THYME

(*Thymus vulgaris*)
This fragrant herb has long been used for medicinal purposes, in cookery, and as an aphrodisiac.

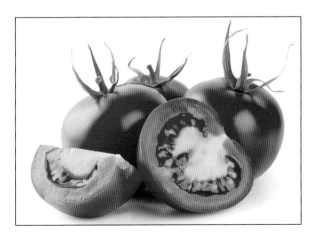

TOMATOES

Tomatoes originate from South America, where they were first cultivated by the Aztecs. Legend has it that sixteenth-century Spanish priests brought tomato seeds to Seville from Peru. They had such a positive effect on those who ate them that the French referred to them as *pommes d'amour*, or "apples of love." Once called Peruvian Apples and grown as purely ornamental plants, tomatoes are now cultivated throughout the world. Together with many other erotic imports, the tomato gained a reputation as an aphrodisiac.

TONGKAT ALI

(*Eurycoma longifolia*)
The tongkat ali tree is one of the most powerful aphrodisiac plants on earth. It is used to treat malaria, high blood pressure, fatigue, and loss of sexual desire. South Asian men enjoy tongkat ali in a plethora of forms, including tea, oil, and supplements. The root is said to contain properties that inhibit aging and it significantly boosts sex drive and function in men and women by increasing testosterone.

TONKA

Tonka is a drug that is obtained from tonquin beans. They have a fragrant aroma, but are bitter to the taste. Tonka is used to flavor foods and is believed to have mild aphrodisiac properties.

TRIBULUS

(*Tribulus terrestris*)
Tribulus terrestris is an Indian plant used in Ayurvedic medicine. Its fruit contains furostanol saponins that are used to treat male genital or urinary problems, low sex drive, and impotence.

TRUFFLES

Truffles are the next most famous aphrodisiac food after oysters. They have an odor reminiscent of the pheromone given off by male pigs. Both the white and black varieties are said to be very potent. The truffle is an edible fungus, indigenous to Europe, known to the Romans as a sexual inducement. Napoleon was advised by one of his generals to eat truffles to increase potency. George IV highly appreciated the virtues of truffles and gave his foreign ministers special directions to forward any superior truffles to the royal kitchen.

Turmeric

(*Curcuma longa*)
Turmeric is a substance derived from the saffron plant. In India it is highly prized as a love stimulant, but is also used as a vaginal douche and in curry.

U

Urad

Urad seeds are a kind of chickpea or gram used in Indian cookery. The Hindu manual *Ananga Ranga* recommends urad for regaining sexual prowess.

V

VALERIAN

(*Valeriana officinalis*)
Valerian is a perennial herb that has long been used as an aphrodisiac. Celtic women wore a sprig of valerian between their breasts to attract lovers. Later it became known as "drunken sailor" and was used by prostitutes. Valerian was used as an aphrodisiac, but these days it is mostly recommended as a sedative.

VANILLA

(*Vanilla planifolia*)
Vanilla is a climbing plant with white flowers that grows in Central America. Vanilla is said to be a potent aphrodisiac and vanilla oil is widely used in perfumery and aromatherapy. The effects of its sensual aroma may be intensified by eating vanilla-flavored confections.

VERVAIN

(*Verbena officinalis*)
This perennial plant grows in hedges and along walls. The pale blue flowers, along with all the other parts of the plant, are used in medicine. It is said the plant would lend the penis the hardness of iron, causing it to be called "ironhard." It is often used in some spells and sex magic.

VUKA-VUKA

First used by Lobengula, the famous African king, vuka-vuka is available for men and women in convenient tea sachets, tablets, capsules, drops, and cream. This is a blend of natural herbs based on a formula used by generations of African men to nurture and enhance sexual responsiveness. It is also recommended for women who need a dietary supplement to boost their stamina and sexual excitement.

W

Walnut

Walnuts are used magically to regain vitality. They are particularly useful to those who have been burning the candle at both ends or are exhausted from sexual overindulgence.

Water lily

Monks, nuns, and clerics of all degrees used to drink daily a concoction consisting of water lilies and the syrup of poppies. This drink was believed to deprive the person of desire for sexual congress.

Wheat

(*Triticum aestivum*)
Wheat is a grain that was first cultivated over six thousand years ago. The medicinally valuable wheat germ has long been used for skin conditions and in massage. There is some investigation on wheat as a love aid due to the high content of vitamin E.

White musali

(*Asparagus adscendens*)
The musali is a long, thin, and thorny plant native to India and the Himalayas. The plant is helpful to the reproductive system and is a useful aphrodisiac that is also an aid to increasing sperm count.

Wild lettuce

(*Lactuca virosa*)
This biennial herb grows in fields and prairies in Europe and North America. A milky sap flows throughout the entire plant and is exuded when it is damaged. This sap was collected by North American Indians, who smoked it as a ritual and sexual stimulant.

Wild lettuce is said to stimulate sexual energy, bring one closer to a higher consciousness, and help aid restful sleep.

WILD YAM

(*Dioscorea villosa*)
Wild yam is a Mexican perennial vine with heart-shaped leaves and small green flowers that is native to North and Central America. It has been used medicinally by North American Indians, Mayans, and Aztecs to relieve pain and to boost libido. It is high in sex hormones, which may account for its ability to boost sex drive in men and women. It is often used as a hormone replacement remedy because of its progesterone-like action in the body.

WINE

A Roman saying held that Venus is lonely without Ceres's bread and Bacchus's wine. However, the Roman epigrammatist Martial stated that too much wine could have the opposite effect, as is the case with any alcohol. Hindu literature too condemns excessive wine drinking in connection with sexual congress.

WITCH HAZEL

(*Hamamelis*)
Witch hazel has, in the past, been considered an erotic inducement if applied externally.

WOODCOCK

Woodcock has long been considered an aphrodisiac and is reputed to boost seminal fluids.

WOOD ROSE

(*Argyreia nervosa*)
Wood rose is a vine found in the dry tropics of Hawaii and South and Southeast Asia. The plant has heart-shaped leaves and funnel-like flowers. The seeds are said to have aphrodisiac qualities and are the main ingredient in the infamous bliss balls.

WORMWOOD

(*Artemisia absinthium*)
Wormwood's leaves and flowers have a very bitter taste and characteristic odor. In the Middle Ages, when sorcery and witchcraft were extensive, spells were frequently cast on a victim's virility. To counteract such a malefic condition, wormwood was used as an antidote. In the nineteenth century, absinthe, a wormwood-based liqueur, was a favorite of the Bohemians. It was said to drive you mad after prolonged use, but had the reputation of an aphrodisiac.

Y

Yage

(*Banisteriopsis caapi*)
Yage is a vine that grows on trees in the northern jungles of South America. The tribes of the South American Orinoco and Amazon basins use yage in their ceremonies. The Tukanoans of Colombia administer the drug to adolescent boys to fortify them for the ritual of entry into manhood. The narcotic drink is a hallucinogen and is used for magic, prophecy, and divination. In Brazil and Peru, yage is used in religious ceremonies, and witch doctors use the plant to diagnose and treat illness and impotence.

Yarrow

(*Achillea millefolium*)
Yarrow is a scented perennial herb used in love magic that was believed to ensure seven years of devotion and faithfulness. North American Indians have used the plant for many years and consider it sacred; it is even consumed as a tea in support of a vision quest. In ancient China, the stem was used in geomancy, especially in the I Ching oracle.

Yerba mate

(*Ilex paraguariensis*)
Yerba mate is a slightly smoky tree that grows only in the rain forest of Paraguay. Sometimes just referred to as mate, its leaves are made into a tea for a nutritional food and stimulant. According to an ancient legend, the sacred formula for preparing the leaf of yerba mate was revealed from Heaven as a reward for faithfulness. It was used to protect against infirmity and is said to incite passion if drunk with a loved one.

YLANG-YLANG

(*Cananga odorata*)
The ylang-ylang tree is ruled by Venus, the goddess of love, and is reputed to make the opposite sex seem more attractive. The tree grows in southern Asia and has long yellow flowers with heart-shaped petals that produce strongly aromatic oil used in massage. The oil can be used to help prevent impotence, frigidity, and depression.

YOHIMBE

(*Pausinystalia yohimbe, Corynanthe yohimbe*)
Yohimbe is a pro-sexual herbal supplement made from the bark of a tall, evergreen tree native to the West African countries of Cameroon, Zaire, and Congo. It is used by many Africans and is one of the most potent aphrodisiac herbs to increase sexual desire, enhance sexual pleasure, boost sexual performance, and treat impotence. Recent research has proved a significant aphrodisiac property in yohimbe when taken as a supplement.

Z

Zallouh

(*Ferulis harmonis*)
Zallouh grows in the mountainous areas of the Middle East. It is a small shrub with thin leaves and tiny white or yellow flowers. The root of the plant has been used as a sex enhancer for thousands of years. Zallouh has a strong tradition of use by men with erectile problems and by men and women with low libido.

Zinc

Zinc is vitally important to healthy sexual functioning. Low zinc levels can contribute to impotence, low sperm count, depression, mood changes, and subfertility. Zinc is very important to the immune system, and prolonged zinc deficiency can lead to real problems.

Appendix 1

A Guide to the Use and Preparation of Herbs, Charms, and Oils as Used in Aphrodisiacs

Charm bags, gris-gris, sachets

The gris-gris, sachet, or charm bag is a form of amulet or talisman that is created to be carried by a person or placed in a certain place in order to gain specific magical effects. It can contain a single object or several, such as herbs, oils, resins, a power object, something personal from the intended recipient, or even written spells.

The making of a charm bag is a magical operation and as such should be carried out in a sacred area. The only difference between a gris-gris and a sachet is that a sachet contains no power objects and is usually sealed and hidden in a particular place.

Elixirs

These are herbs infused in either alcohol or a mixture of wine and alcohol. Sometimes instructions are given in the text for elixirs from certain plants detailing the method or brewing or type of alcohol. These are generally taken a drop or two at a time or as a drink in wine, spirits, or mead. But, as with every new substance that you decide to take internally, exercise caution and be very sure that the substances you have chosen to use are not hallucinogenic or poisonous. It is also possible to make elixirs from gemstones, which are used to imbibe the power or properties of the chosen gemstone.

INCENSE

Incense is a substance that makes fragrant smoke. The easiest way to make your own incense is to use charcoal disks containing saltpeter. These discs must be used on a heat-resistant surface or in a proper censer, as they generate a lot of heat. Many substances that can be used singly or in combination to make incenses are mentioned in this book, but the easiest way to use incense is to buy ready-made incense sticks.

OIL OR PERFUME

There are two forms of oils that are primarily used in aphrodisiac preparations or love enchantments: pure essential oils of the plant or resin and infused oils. Essential oils are basically the pure essence that is pressed from the herb and should contain no adulterants. Infused oils are made from neutral vegetable oils that have had the appropriate herb, flower, or resin placed in them to infuse their perfume in the carrier oil. Making your own infused oils can be a good way of obtaining substances that are not generally available or are prohibitively expensive.

OINTMENT OR BALMS

Ointments are a solid way of using and storing herbs and are usually made to rub into the skin.

PHILTERS AND POWDERS

A philter is a drink that is supposed to excite sexual love in the drinker or any powdered herb that can be taken in minuscule doses. A powder is not always taken internally, but can instead be sprinkled onto clothes, around the home, or in a place where someone or something will come into contact with it. Philters can also be used in this way.

POTPOURRI

A potpourri is a simple, modern way to use herbs for ritualistic purposes. Take a selection of herbs, spices, and oils for the purpose you require and make a fragrant mixture. Leave this mixture in a bowl in your room to create an appropriate atmosphere. Mixes can be purchased now quite easily, but experiment and make up your own mixes from dried flowers, pinecones, bits of bark, fruit peel, or shells.

POTIONS, BREWS, TEAS, INFUSIONS, OR DECOCTIONS

A standard brew or infusion for the majority of herbs is made from 0.8 ounces dried herb or 2.5 ounces fresh herb in 17 ounces of boiling water. The brew can be taken hot or cooled either in the refrigerator or freezer. Standard dosage is half a cup a day.

A tisane, or herb tea, also known as a brew or potion, is a weaker infusion made by putting 1 teaspoon of dried herb into a mug of boiling water. A decoction is usually made from 1 ounce of the root of a plant or wood added to 1 pint of boiling water. Simmer until the liquid has reduced by half. This method is used only on tough substances since prolonged boiling will often destroy properties of normal herbs. Therefore use a tisane or infusion unless otherwise stated.

SMOKING AND SMUDGING

There are two types of smoking involved in sexual ritual practices. One method is smoking an herb in a pipe or rolled into a cigarette and inhaling the smoke as one would use tobacco. The other way to use smoke is to cleanse the body, a room, a house, or magical equipment. This process is often called smudging and may also be used to imbue something with the powers of a particular herb, usually sage.

The theory behind smudging is that the smoke attaches itself to negative energy, which it removes as it clears, releasing it into another space to be regenerated. The skillful and proper use of sage could help in warding and banishing ceremonies as well. You can, and should, regularly smudge your meditation area, your altar if you have one, and any object that you use for healing before and after use. This ensures that the healing object will be able to do its job with the least amount of interference from dead energy that may be holding it back.

STEAM

Steaming is a good way of using the perfume of herbs without burning them. Traditionally, herbs are placed in water in a cauldron, which is either suspended above a fire or stood at one edge among the embers. As the water comes to a boil, it gives off a perfumed steam that can be inhaled or used to cleanse the body for divination or the creation of a romantic or calming atmosphere. Oil evaporators are more often used today, which necessitate water and a few drops of essential oil being put in a bowl over a lit candle. Essential oils can also be put in your bath or left in bowls of warm water to scent the air.

WASH WATERS

Wash waters are diluted infusions of herbs that are used to bathe in or wash large areas. Wash waters are in general used for psychic cleansing, consecration, and the banishment of unwanted vibrations, but they can also be used to attract certain influences or set moods.

Bibliography

Anand, Margot. *The Art of Sexual Ecstasy: The Path of Sacred Sexuality for Western Lovers.* New York: Thorsons Publishers, 1991.

Bhagwan, Dash and Suhasini Ramaswamy. *Indian Aphrodisiacs.* New Delhi: Roli Books, Lustre Press, 2001.

Brewer, Sarah. *Increase Your Sex Drive: The Amazing Power of Supplements, Herbs and Instant Aphrodisiacs.* New York: Thorsons Publishers, 1999.

Brook, Jasmine. *Spells for Love and Success.* Wigston: Abbeydale Press, 2001.

Catty, Suzanne. *Hydrosols: The Next Aromatherapy.* Rochester: Healing Arts Press, 2001.

Chia, Mantak with Michael Winn. *Taoist Secrets of Love: Cultivating Male Sexual Energy.* Santa Fe: Aurora Press, 1984.

Davenport, John. *Aphrodisiacs and Love Stimulants with Other Chapters on the Secrets of Venus.* London: Luxor Press, 1965.

De Luca, Diana. *Botanica Erotica: Arousing Body, Mind, and Spirit.* Rochester: Healing Arts Press, 1998.

Devi, Kamala. *The Eastern Way of Love: Tantric Sex and Erotic Mysticism.* New York: Simon & Schuster, 1985.

Eason, Cassandra. *A Magical Guide to Love and Sex.* London: Piatkus, 2000.

Golden, Arthur. *Memoirs of a Geisha.* London: Vintage, 1998.

Harvey, Karen, ed. *The Kiss in History*. Manchester: Manchester University Press, 2005.

Kilham, Chris. *Hot Plants: Nature's Proven Sex Boosters for Men and Women*. New York: St. Martin's Press, 2004.

Millar, Elisabeth. *Releasing Aphrodite: Aromatic Aphrodisiacs for Love and Romance*. Hove: Capricorn Press, 2006.

Morris, Desmond. *The Naked Woman*. London: Vintage, 2004.

Nefzawi, Sheik, trans. Sir Richard Burton, ed. Alan Hull Walton. *The Perfumed Garden*. London: Grafton Books, 1986.

Ratsch, Christian. *Plants of Love: The History of Aphrodisiacs and a Guide to Their Identification and Use*. London: Ten Speed Press, 1997.

Runcie, James. *The Discovery of Chocolate*. New York: HarperCollins, 2001.

Sellar, Wanda. *The Directory of Essential Oils*. London: The C. W. Daniel Company, 1992.

Sempers, Chris. *The Magical Herbal Spellbook*. London: Corvus Books, 1998.

Simons, G. L. *The Illustrated Book of Sexual Records*. London: Virgin Books, 1982.

Tisserand, Maggie. *Essence of Love: Fragrance, Aphrodisiacs, and Aromatherapy for Lovers*. New York: HarperCollins, 1994.

Ward, Tim. *Savage Breast: One Man's Search for the Goddess*. Hants: O Books, 2006.

Wedeck, Harry E. *A Dictionary of Aphrodisiacs*. New York: M. Evans & Company, Inc., 1992.

Glossary

Adrenergic:	Pertains to that transmission of information through the nervous system that is moderated by adrenaline
Anal aphrodisiac:	A substance that stimulates the erogenous zones on the anus
Anaphrodisiac:	Suppressing the desire for sex
Androsterone:	A male sexual hormone
Anomaly:	Deviating from the norm; malformation
Anthelmintic:	A drug that expels or kills parasitic worms
Anti-aphrodisiac:	Suppressing the desire for sex
Anticholinergic:	A substance that blocks the formation of the neurotransmitters acetylcholine and choline; many substances traditionally used as aphrodisiacs have this effect
Antisyphilitic:	An agent used to combat syphilis
Arteriosclerosis:	A condition characterized by a thickening or hardening of the arteries
Asarone:	Asarum camphor, a plant substance that is transformed into a psychedelic and aphrodisiac phenethylamine
Astringent:	Having the property of constricting body tissues

Ayurveda:	The ancient Indian science of life healing and medicine
Biogenic:	Produced as a result of life processes
Buttons:	Dried slices cut from a peyote cactus
Cunnilingus:	Oral stimulation of the female genitalia
Decoction:	The boiling of herbs and drugs in order to produce a concentrate
Dildo:	A synthetic penis used for self-gratification
Diuretic:	An agent that causes urination or stimulates kidney activity
Dysmenorrhea:	Painful or difficult menstruation
Emmenagogue:	Herbs that induce menstruation
Endemic:	Native; limited to an area
Enema:	A liquid preparation intended for injection into the rectum or lower intestinal tract
Enzyme:	A biocatalyst that affects metabolic processes in an organism
Ephedrine:	A plant substance used as the model for amphetamine
Estrogen:	A female sexual hormone
Fellatio:	The oral stimulation of the penis
Flagellation:	The act of sexual stimulation by means of whipping
Frigidity:	Lacking friendliness or sexual enthusiasm
Fumigation:	The ritual use of smoke to purify or perfume a person, object, or place
Galactagogue:	An agent that induces the flow of milk
Geomancy:	Soothsaying, divining, or interpreting objects

Geriatric:	A branch of medicine that deals with the problems and diseases of old age
Gonorrhea:	A sexually transmitted disease
Herpes:	A sexually transmitted disease
Hedonistic:	Relating to pleasure
Hepatitis:	Inflammation of the liver
Homeopathy:	A system of medical practice that is based upon the focused administration of extremely minute concentrations of drugs and plant materials
Hydrosol:	A flower water, such as rosewater, frequently a byproduct of the manufacture of essential oils
Ibogaine:	A plant substance that has anti-depressive, monoamine oxidase–inhibiting, psychedelic, and aphrodisiac effects
Irritation:	Inflammation or soreness in a part of the body
Ithyphallic:	An artistic representation of an erect phallus
Lactation:	The process of milk coming from the breast
Libations:	Sacrificial rites in temples, usually involving liquids like wine and alcohol
Luteinizing hormone:	A gonadotropic HVL hormone that stimulates the intestinal cells
Maceration:	An extract of a drug made at room temperature by steeping some solvent like alcohol in water
Menorrhagia:	Abnormally heavy menstrual bleeding
Mycelium:	The subterranean root mass of a fungus
Neuralgia:	The acute pain in an area innervated by a sensory nerve
Neurotransmitter:	A chemical information carrier in the nervous system

Orchitis: Inflammation of a testis

Pruritus: Itching pertaining to the anus or the genitals

Priapic: Pertaining to the ithyphallic God of fertility, Priapus

Priapism: An abnormal, pathological stiffening of the penis that can result in damage to the corpora cavernosa

Prolactin: A hormone that induces lactation produced in the interior lobe of the pituitary

Psilocin: A psychedelic substance of the tryptamine group found in certain fungi

Satyr: Lusty mythological figure who is one of the followers of Dionysus or Bacchus

Testosterone: A male sexual hormone

Tincture: A preparation produced from fresh or dried plants by means of extraction

Tonic: An agent that invigorates or strengthens

Urtication: A treatment employing stinging nettles and an old remedy for invigorating one's sexual life and combating impotence